THE
BENZODIAZEPINES

SECOND EDITION

THE BENZODIAZEPINES

USE, OVERUSE, MISUSE, ABUSE

by

John Marks
MA MD FRCP FRCPsych

Fellow, Tutor and Director of Medical Studies
Girton College, Cambridge

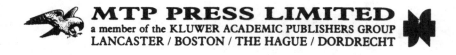

MTP PRESS LIMITED
a member of the KLUWER ACADEMIC PUBLISHERS GROUP
LANCASTER / BOSTON / THE HAGUE / DORDRECHT

Published in the UK and Europe by
MTP Press Limited
Falcon House
Lancaster, England

British Library Cataloguing in Publication Data

Marks, John, 1924–
    The benzodiazepines: use, overuse, misuse, abuse.—2nd ed.
    1. Benzodiazepines 2. Drug abuse
    I. Title
    615'.7882   RM666.B42

    ISBN 0–85200–870–8

Published in the USA by
MTP Press
A division of Kluwer Boston Inc
190 Old Derby Street
Hingham, MA 02043, USA

Library of Congress Cataloging in Publication Data

Marks, John, 1924–
    The benzodiazepines: use, overuse, misuse, abuse.

    Bibliography: p.
    Includes index.
    1. Benzodiazepine abuse. I. Title.
RC568.B45M37 1985   616.86'3   85–10581
ISBN 0–85200–870–8

Typesetting by Titus Wilson & Son Ltd., Kendal, Cumbria
Printed in Great Britain by
Butler & Tanner Ltd, Frome and London

Contents

Preface   vii

Glossary   viii

Part I

General considerations

1   The general problem of dependence and abuse   3

Part II

Benzodiazepine dependence and abuse

2   Animal studies of dependence liability   11

3   Experimental studies on benzodiazepine dependence in humans   18

4   Patterns of benzodiazepine dependence   27

5   The pathophysiological mechanisms of benzodiazepine dependence   30

6   Description of the benzodiazepine withdrawal reaction   33

7   Literature appraisal – benzodiazepine dependence during therapeutic use   39

8   Benzodiazepine 'street scene' abuse   49

Part III

Significance of benzodiazepine dependence within the community

9   Medical aspects   61
10 Social aspects   79
11 Legal aspects   92
12 Consideration of long-term use   100
13 Practical aspects of benzodiazepine use   106

Part IV

Conclusions

14 Summary and conclusions   113

Appendix 1 Case reports   115
Appendix 2 Studies on the incidence of withdrawal reactions with benzodiazepines at therapeutic dosage   128
References   135
Index   159

Preface

In 1978 I wrote a monograph on the overuse, misuse and abuse of the benzodiazepines based on my experience within the Roche organization during the development and marketing of the benzodiazepines, and subsequently within academic medical practice. This monograph, *inter alia*, reviewed the published cases of reputed benzodiazepine dependence from 1960 to mid 1976 and attempted to assess the risk of dependence and abuse.

Since 1978 medical and lay interest in the question of the benzodiazepines has continued. Some of the lay media comment has been emotional and inaccurate and has led to medical problems, though it is clear that the overall interest and discussion of the issues has been beneficial for good medical practice.

The 1978 monograph stressed that high dosage and simultaneous ingestion of other substances of dependence were the main factors in the genesis of dependence. Since then it has become clear that while these are important factors, dependence can occur at normal therapeutic dosage.

Other changes that have occurred since 1978 have been the large number of new benzodiazepines that are available; the overall fall in the use of these substances in most countries and developments in our knowledge of cellular mechanism of actions of the benzodiazepines.

In consequence of these various factors a substantial revision of the monograph appeared necessary and this I have done. As on the previous occasion I have benefited greatly from discussions that I have had with psychiatrists, pharmacologists and legislators in many parts of the world. I should like to acknowledge especially the help given me by John Ward and Jean Kilshaw. However, the interpretation and any errors of commission and omisson are mine alone.

Cambridge, March 1985   JOHN MARKS

Glossary

Abstinence syndrome The syndrome which occurs in drug-dependent people when the drug is withheld. It usually involves both physical and psychological manifestations, the nature of which varies with the drug on which dependence exists. It is also termed withdrawal reaction (q.v.) or withdrawal syndrome.

Addiction A term which is still widely used but which is variously understood and defined by physicians, sociologists and lawyers. It should be discarded for scientific literature and replaced by the term dependence (q.v.) as defined by the World Health Organization.

Crutch phenomenon The reaction to some drugs (e.g. glyceryl trinitrate, psychotropics) which is akin to psychological dependence (q.v.) but in which the patient feels the need to *carry* the drugs in case problems arise.

Drug Any substance which when taken into the living organism may modify one or more of its functions.

Drug abuse Persistent or sporadic excessive drug use inconsistent with or unrelated to acceptable medical practice; cf. 'Misuse' (q.v.). The term abuse covers a wide range of different types of inappropriate use.

Drug dependence A state, psychic and sometimes also physical, which results from the interaction between a living organism and a drug, which is characterized by behavioural and other responses that always include a compulsion to take the drug on a continuous or periodic basis in order to experience its psychic effects and sometimes to avoid the discomfort of its absence. Tolerance may be present.

Misuse Medical or lay use of a drug for a disease state not considered to be appropriate by the majority. This has a close relationship with the term 'abuse' but the latter can probably best be considered in the more general context of 'affect modification' for personal gratification, whereas the former implies an attempted therapeutic effect, however misguided.

Overuse Excessive medical or lay use of a drug, in terms of length of therapy or severity of disorder treated, for diseases in which there is accepted evidence of therapeutic effect.

Physical dependence The drug, or one or more of its metabolites, has become necessary for the continued functioning of certain body processes. This creates in the dependent person on withdrawal of the drug true physically determined and clinically recognizable signs (the abstinence syndrome – q.v.). These are usually heavily overlaid with psychologically determined symptoms and often manifestations of the disease for which the drug was originally taken.

Pseudo withdrawal reaction A reaction which mimics the abstinence syndrome (q.v.) except that the drug has not actually been withdrawn. It stems from an expectation of problems generated by media anecdotal reports.

Psychoactive substance Any substance which influences mental processes.

Psychological dependence This involves purely emotional components with no physical signs on withdrawal. It runs at one end of the spectrum from the degrees of subjective pleasure or relief of symptoms that are experienced from the drug, through the emotional drives that lead the person to persist in its use, to the change in lifestyle, behaviour and personal involvement where the life pattern revolves around drug taking and the company of others similarly involved. At this extreme the drug use provides a total deviant career often lived as a member of a subculture of drug users alienated by behaviour or law from normal society. It can be regarded as a pharmacological, an anxiety avoidance or a positive operant conditioning response to the drug itself.

Psychotropic substance Any substance which, according to WHO definition, influences mental processes and on which dependence occurs. In general parlance it has been used extensively for any medicine for mental disorders but in view of the WHO definition this use should probably be dropped.

Rebound phenomenon An overreaction of the body processes immediately after suppression by drug activity is removed. It is a common reaction to many drugs.

Tolerance (sometimes referred to as '**acquired tolerance**') The need to employ increasing doses of a drug in order to produce the same effect. This may depend on altered sensitivity of the cell receptor, on increased rates of metabolism of the drug or changes in cell transmitter substances.

Withdrawal reaction (also called '**withdrawal syndrome**') The reaction which occurs when a drug, given for some time, is suddenly withdrawn. It includes the abstinence syndrome (q.v.) with drug dependence; return of the disorder previously controlled by the treatment; pseudo withdrawal reaction (q.v.); crutch phenomenon (q.v.); rebound phenomenon (q.v.).

Part I
General considerations

1
The General Problem of Dependence and Abuse

That humanity at large will ever be able to dispense with Artificial Paradises seems very unlikely. Most men and women lead lives at the worst so painful, at the best so monotonous, poor and limited that the urge to escape, the longing to transcend themselves if only for a few moments, is and has always been one of the principal appetites of the soul. Art and religion, carnivals and saturnalia, dancing and listening to oratory – all these have served, in H. G. Wells' phrase, as 'doors in the wall'. And for private, everyday use, there have always been chemical intoxicants. All the vegetable sedatives and narcotics, all the euphorics that grow on trees, the hallucinogens that ripen in berries or can be squeezed from roots – all, without exception, have been known and systematically used by human beings from time immemorial. And to these natural modifiers of consciousness modern science has added its quota of synthetics – chloral, for example, and benzedrine, the bromides, and the barbiturates.

Most of these modifiers of consciousness cannot now be taken except under doctor's orders, or else illegally and at considerable risk. For unrestricted use the West has permitted only alcohol and tobacco. All the other chemical 'doors in the wall' are labelled 'dope', and their unauthorized takers are 'fiends' (Huxley, 1959).

There is scarcely any agent which can be taken into the body to which some individuals will not get a reaction satisfactory or pleasurable to them, persuading them to continue its use even to the point of abuse (Eddy *et al.*, 1965).

At the present time, indeed for many centuries past, there can be few people throughout the world who do not 'overuse', 'misuse' or 'abuse' some drug. For many the drugs that are 'overused' are caffeine (from tea

3

or coffee), nicotine (from tobacco) or alcohol (from beer, wine or spirits), all socially accepted normal ingredients of everyday life in most communities. For a smaller group the 'misuse' concerns commonly prescribed medical substances, e.g. barbiturates, amphetamines. For an even smaller group there is the less socially acceptable or frankly unacceptable 'abuse' of specific substances such as solvents, morphine and related analgesics, cannabis, or hallucinogens.

Each of these substances is usually taken to provide some form of positive pleasure or to relieve stress, anxiety, depression or pain.

Much of this field of study is still covered with confusion, not only because the socially acceptable practices of one generation or community are the legally enforceable abuses of another, but because much of the terminology that has been employed has become subject to lack of general agreement.

The term that is still in the widest general use is 'addiction', but because of the differences that exist in its understanding there is a growing tendency to use the word 'dependence' and to adopt the World Health Organization's definitions (WHO, 1950). The basic terms are 'drug', 'drug abuse' and 'drug dependence' and the World Health Organization's definitions for these terms have already been given in the glossary.

The WHO recommendation (WHO, 1964) is that when drug dependence is being discussed the type should be specified because there is considerable variation in the possible features, in their intensity and in their importance to the individual and to society. The question of types is discussed later (p. 7) and as more studies are undertaken the recognized number of types is extended. To these basic WHO definitions it is convenient to add certain others, namely 'misuse', 'overuse' and 'tolerance' and these terms are also defined in the glossary. These definitions will be used in this monograph to minimize confusion.

The World Health Organization definition of dependence can with advantage be elaborated to include the concept of physical and psychological dependence (see glossary), though in many instances this distinction appears to be somewhat arbitrary.

One further term which can cause confusion in its usage is 'psychotropic'. By basic definition any substance that can lead to dependence must be psychoactive, i.e. alter the mental processes. Such substances, and particularly those used for therapy of mental disorders, have been termed 'psychotropics' or 'psychotropic substances'. However, the UNO definition reserves the term 'psychotropic' for a substance which leads to dependence (UNO, 1971a) and the term psychoactive is therefore probably more appropriate as the general term for the group.

A BROADER CONCEPT OF 'PSYCHOTROPICS'

It has already been stressed (p. 3) that there are few of us who do not resort to some form of 'drug' (taking that term in its wide WHO definition), in a manner that must come broadly within the format of psychological dependence. That is to say there is an unnatural drive towards the 'drug' for a pleasure-seeking goal. For most of us the 'drug' concerned is one of the socially accepted beverages; tea, coffee or alcohol, although even within these socially accepted drinks a spectrum of dependence becomes immediately apparent with alcohol at the high-risk end but with caffein-ism also recognized as a problem (Greden, 1974; Gilbert, 1976; Greden et al., 1981).

Each of these substances can be classed as a psychotropic 'drug' by the UN/WHO definition, for there is a mood change as a result of its ingestion, and some measure of dependence.

It is then important to realize that the concept of psychotropic can be extended beyond the realm of drugs, for a broad range of human activities can be used to produce a mood change. What is then apparent is that on each of these some measure of psychological dependence occurs assayed in terms of an unnatural drive towards that pleasure-seeking goal. This may just consist of the need for the cup of tea on waking up; the obsessional completion of *The Times* crossword; the cultivation of prize blooms or vegetables; the irrational drive to watch some form of sport on a regular basis. It extends in well over 50% of the populations of developed countries into the socially acceptable but true 'addictions' of smoking, drinking and gambling.

Peer and priest, senator and serf, doctor and dustman alike experience one or more excessive pleasure-seeking drives. We should consider each of these activities within a wider concept of 'psychotropics' and perhaps speak of those that are socially acceptable as the 'social psychotropics'.

However, the concept of social acceptability immediately raises a value-judgement. Within the group of the psychotropics such a judgement is difficult for there are no scientifically definable borders or limits between the various grades of dependence that exist – rather we should view the whole range of psychotropics as a spectrum (Figure 1). At one end of the scale are the commonplace socially unacceptable patterns of those dependent, for example, on heroin. But how do we assign a rating order for the intermediate dependences? It is difficult to do so scientific-ally, for we are biased by the social fashions of our culture, nation and age and by our own predilections and aversions. But even if we establish a rating order, it is very difficult to define the border between acceptability and non-acceptability without value-judgements subject to bias. The United Nations' Convention (UNO, 1971a) adopts the concept of 'public health and social problems' when the need for action is considered.

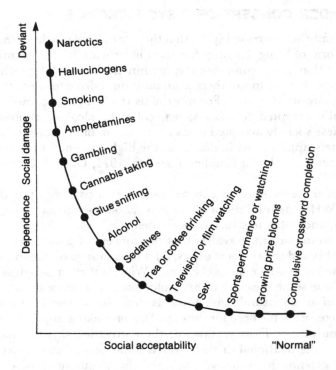

Figure 1 The broad concept of psychotropics as the range of pleasure-giving activities of the community for which some measure of unnatural drive (or dependence) exists. Examination shows that the rating order of the individual activities must represent the bias of the author. While the extremes can be labelled 'Deviant' and 'Normal' with accuracy and ease, the limit of social acceptability depends upon a value judgement influenced by political, social and individual factors

This view of drug misuse as an example of a broad range of pleasure-seeking drives has been denied by others (Keup, 1982), but it is still regarded as a useful working hypothesis which explains the wide-ranging activity of pleasure-seeking within the community. It stresses that drug misuse involves not only factors related to the substance itself, but also to the host and the environment (Stepney, 1980).

Just as normal levels of anxiety can be an important drive for the examinee or athlete, and morbid anxiety can destroy the ability, so can nearly all these pleasure-seeking drives stimulate work for good or evil. The social object should be to encourage that for good and attempt to remove the component that brings evil. Education (p. 5) will help this, but legislation rarely does so and should be reserved for those activities where the dangers to society as a whole are greatest. This is considered in more detail on pp. 7 *et seq.*

Thus the problem of dependence on drugs, the topic that is of prime interest to us, must be viewed not in isolation but as part of the wide realm of a full spectrum of 'psychotropics', many of which can be 'overused' or indeed 'abused', and which give rise to dependence.

Specifically we are concerned with the benzodiazepines, a group of therapeutic substances on which dependence and abuse can occur. This monograph considers benzodiazepine dependence and abuse and the factors that influence it. It attempts to put the dependence and abuse in clinical perspective and to define how the benzodiazepines should be used in clinical practice to reduce the risks while maintaining the therapeutic benefits.

TYPES OF DRUG DEPENDENCE

The WHO expert committee has recognized that different groups of drugs produce different types of dependence and that the type should be specified. The currently accepted types, the main classes of drugs involved and the clinical characteristics of the dependence are shown in Table 1. Apart from noting the great variety of types that are now recognized, the majority of classes can be ignored for the purpose of the present monograph and attention can be concentrated on the groups of ethanol and barbiturate/sedative. There are still divergent opinions on whether they should be grouped together – for both show psychological and physical dependence with virtually identical withdrawal reactions – or whether they should be separated. In favour of their being put into a single group is the extensive cross-tolerance that can occur among drugs with similar actions, regardless of chemical structure, and the partial effectiveness of one group in ameliorating the withdrawal efffects of the other.

Thus, for example, severe ethanol withdrawal reactions can be prevented by barbiturates (Essig et al., 1969), phenothiazines (Sereny and Kalant, 1965), benzodiazepines (Sereny and Kalant, 1965; Kaim, 1973), chloral hydrate and paraldehyde (Kaim et al., 1969). Conversely ethanol is partially effective in the prevention of barbiturate withdrawal phenomena (Frazer et al., 1957). Such sedatives, however, have no specific effect on the morphine-type withdrawal syndromes, although other members of that group can cross-substitute (e.g. methadone for morphine) – and sedatives can reduce the severity of some of the manifestations.

Despite this evidence of cross-substitution between ethanol and the barbiturate/sedatives it is probably wiser to regard them as separate groups at the present time. Benzodiazepine dependence is clearly recognized as falling within the sedative type, though the incidence and severity differs substantially from that of some other sedatives (e.g. methaqualone).

7

Table 1 Dependence types that are currently recognized and their clinical features

Type	Representative drugs	Psychological dependence	Clinical features of abstinence
Morphine type	Morphine diamorphine methadone pethidine, etc.	Severe rapid psychological dependence with initial euphoria but later passivity and inertia Tolerance ++	Restlessness, rubbing the face and body, irritability, yawning, salivation, apprehension, nausea, vomiting, abdominal cramps, tremors, joint pains, running eyes and nose, diarrhoea and in later stages elevated blood pressure, raised blood sugar and spontaneous ejaculation or orgasm
Cocaine type	Cocaine	Severe psychological dependence, mainly stimulant No true tolerance	No physical dependence
Cannabis type	Tetrahydrocannabinol	Severe psychological dependence with deteriorated social behaviour, apathy, indolence and inertia No tolerance	No physical dependence
Amphetamine type	Amphetamine and related phenylethylamines	Severe psychological dependence with excitement, restless irritability, repetitive overactivity and hallucinations Tolerance ++	? physical dependence – see under psychological dependence
Hallucinogen type	LSD psilocybin mescaline khat	Psychological dependence with emotional lability, hallucinations and morbid deterioration of social behaviour Tolerance develops to most	? physical dependence
Solvents	Ether 'Glue'	Psychological dependence	Can lead on to abuse of other substances
Ethanol type	All alcoholic beverages methylated spirit	Psychological dependence of varying severity and rapidity of development. There is variation in early behaviour with later gross deterioration of social behaviour Tolerance +	Anxiety, sleeplessness, coarse tremors, weakness, abdominal cramps, hallucinations, disorientation, convulsions
Barbiturate/ sedative type	Barbiturates glutethimide meprobamate methaqualone	Psychological dependence which varies in severity and rapidity of development between drugs and between patients Varying degrees of deterioration of social behaviour Tolerance common to most drugs	Anxiety, insomnia, anorexia, nausea, vomiting, muscle twitching, delirium and convulsions
Tobacco	Cigarettes, etc.	Psychological dependence severe Tolerance present	EEG and sleep changes. Reduced performance in some psychomotor tests
Caffeine	Tea Coffee	? mild psychological dependence Some tolerance	No physical dependence

Part II
Benzodiazepine dependence and abuse

2
Animal studies of dependence liability

Animal models are available for the study of both psychological and physical dependence of sedative type.

PSYCHOLOGICAL DEPENDENCE STUDIES

The most important animal model for the study of psychological dependence is the operant model using a response produced by the automatic intravenous or intragrastic self-administration of the drug of the type that was originally used for opiate studies (see for example WHO, 1964, 1975, 1978). The oral and intravenous routes each have their own particular advantages and limitations, as well as those shared by both.

Intravenous self-administration studies

The animal is trained to self-administer the drug solution through an indwelling cannula by pressing a bar which activates the injection pump. The literature, particularly that relating to opiates, has been extensively reviewed. (Weeks, 1962; Thompson and Pickens, 1969; Deneau, 1969; Schuster and Thompson, 1969; Thompson and Pickens, 1970) and shows that different groups of drugs have different potencies as operant reinforcers. Thus opiates, amphetamines and cocaine are highly potent; ethanol and barbiturates moderately so; and mescaline and phenothiazines relatively ineffective. Not all animals of the same species respond to reinforcement in the same way but some develop drug intake patterns which, like those of dependent humans, lead to physical illness and gross withdrawal reactions.

The study of intravenous drug administration is undertaken by examining the rate at which some automatically recorded response such as pressing a lever is made. In order to demonstrate reinforcement by a

11

drug, the response level with the drug should be found to be above that maintained by the vehicle used for its solution.

Many different drug self-administration procedures have been used. The simplest is that in which each response produces a drug infusion – designated as fixed ratio 1 response, with unlimited drug access. Access to the drug may be limited to certain experimental periods during the day. Other more complex techniques and schedules have been devised but few have been used for the benzodiazepines.

The fixed ratio 1 schedule with unlimited drug access may appear to be the most simple, and most easily interpreted. However, it is not always the most effective. For example with the narcotics (Werner *et al.*, 1976) or stimulants (Pickens and Harris, 1968), very low rates of response can be maintained under fixed ratio 1 schedules with continuous access, while under other conditions the same animal may respond at a much higher rate (Kelleher, 1976). The interval between injections is an important factor, and when the rate at which injections are permitted to occur is limited, the response rates are often higher.

The standard of the publications in this area is extremely variable and it is sometimes difficult to interpret the results. There is often a lack of information about the dose per injection or the type of vehicle and details concerning the response rate to the vehicle itself. When attempting to interpret the results it must be remembered that the drugs themselves have pharmacological activities in addition to any reinforcing effect. Such pharmacological activities will vary with the dose administered and with the rate and frequency of administration. Hence variability of response may not depend only on the reinforcing effect of the drug.

The majority of the animal studies on benzodiazepine self-administration have used rhesus monkeys, and the drug which has been studied most extensively has been diazepam.

Yanagita and Takahashi (1973) reported that intravenous injections of 0.4 mg/kg per injection diazepam maintained the response above vehicle levels in three out of the four monkeys. Other studies have reported that diazepam does not maintain a response when administered intravenously (e.g. Hackett and Hall, 1977).

An alternative type of study has compared the substitution of benzodiazepines or the vehicle in animals already maintaining self-administration of either cocaine or codeine. Most of these studies have confirmed moderate reinforcing properties of the different benzodiazepines (Hoffmeister, 1977; Griffiths *et al.*, 1981), but Hackett and Hall (1977) could not demonstrate such a reinforcing effect in such studies.

Hence, while it appears that animals will self-administer benzodiazepines by the intravenous route rather more frequently than the vehicle, the results are not striking or consistent.

Oral and intragastric ingestion studies

In such studies the drug is administered in solution or suspension orally (in drinking water or food) or through an intragastric cannula. The oral or intragastric administration of benzodiazepines appears to be more relevant to human therapy, and has been more extensively studied in animals. Most of the studies of oral ingestion of benzodiazepines have used rats as subjects, but other animal species have also been investigated.

When both water and a benzodiazepine solution are continuously available there is no preference for the latter (Kamano and Arp, 1965; Harris et al., 1968; Amit and Cohen, 1974; Yanaura and Tagashira, 1975). To overcome this problem and to induce greater drug intake various techniques have been used. For example some studies have assessed the development of preference when just drug-laced water or drug-laced food were available (Harris et al., 1968; Stolerman et al., 1971; Yanaura and Tagashira, 1975). None of these studies showed the development of preference for drug-laced food or fluid following periods of forced consumption of either chlordiazepoxide or diazepam.

Various other techniques have been used to try to increase the amount of intake. In a study in which the animals were deprived of fluid for a day and then allowed access to a diazepam solution (Walton and Deutsch, 1978), the volume of fluid intake did not differ from the control level on days when water laced with diazepam was given. However as the diazepam concentration increased, the amount of drug consumed in that constant volume of course increased. There was a progressive decrease in the consumption in a similar study with chlordiazepoxide solution in which the bitter taste was not masked (Wolf et al., 1978). Electrical stimulation of the lateral hypothalamus was ineffective in inducing the consumption of diazepam solution (Amit and Cohen, 1974) while stressful painful electric shocks did not induce a significant consumption of a chlordiazepoxide solution (Kamano and Arp, 1965).

Sanger (1977), with a schedule-induced fluid intake, found the highest intake in a group on 0.1 mg/ml chlordiazepoxide, but the control water group was higher than fluids containing 0.2–0.4 mg/ml chlordiazepoxide. Griffiths and Ator (1981) suggested that this represented a reinforcing effect, despite the fact that Sanger had previously shown that chlordiazepoxide itself induced increased fluid intake, and that Jacquet and Stokes (1975) could not induce significant chlordiazepoxide preference with a schedule-induced model.

Harris et al. (1968) used a more complicated technique. Food-deprived rats were food-reinforced to drink a drug solution. A meprobamate-laced solution produced a higher level of intake than chlordiazepoxide-laced fluid. Further studies in baboons have been undertaken by Ator and Griffiths (1982). There was a small preference for triazolam over the vehicle solution, but much clearer drug preferences with methohexital. Hence, overall, the results with oral administration (as opposed to intragastric) do not show a strong benzodiazepine-reinforcing effect, but this might be influenced by the bitter taste of these substances.

Intragastric administration of benzodiazepines has been studied by Yanagita and Takahashi (1973), Gotestam (1973), Weaver *et al.* (1975), Yanagita *et al.* (1975b–e, 1976), Yanagita and Kiyohara (1976), Davis *et al.* (1978), Altschuler and Phillips (1978), Yanagita *et al.* (1981b), Yanagita and Kato (1982).

The exact methods and benzodiazepine used have varied from one study to another. The intragastric studies have at best produced equivocal data concerning the reinforcing effects of the drug. The effects are often not supported by clear differentiation between drug and vehicle response rates and the results may be misleading by averaging over an excessive time period during which rates of response were progressively decreasing. Moreover the results show great variability both within and between subjects. Even zopiclone, which has a non-benzodiazepine structure but is known to act through benzodiazepine receptors, is readily self-administered intragastrically by monkeys (Yanagita, 1983).

Hence, taken overall, we may conclude that in these animal experiments it is difficult to induce amounts of benzodiazepine self-administration sufficient to produce significant degrees of intoxication. The best evidence for any reinforcing effect in animal self-administration comes from those studies that have used short-acting benzodiazepines (Lukas and Griffiths, 1982a). On the other hand, comparison in animal studies suggests that the barbiturates of short or intermediate duration of action are usually more effective reinforcers than any of the benzodiazepines. In direct preference studies where the rate of response is used as a measure of the strength of the reinforcing effects, barbiturates with an equivalent duration of action tend to show a much stronger reinforcing effect than benzodiazepines (Griffiths *et al.*, 1981).

PHYSICAL DEPENDENCE STUDIES

The studies of physical dependence on benzodiazepines in animals have been of two types. The first examines the capacity of the benzodiazepines to produce a withdrawal state as a consequence of chronic administration followed by abstinence. These are the primary dependence studies. In recent studies of this type the administration of a benzodiazepine antagonist (Ro 15–1788) has been used to precipitate the withdrawal effect in animals (Lukas and Griffiths, 1982b,c; Rosenberg and Chiu, 1982; Cumin *et al.*, 1982; McNicholas and Martin, 1982a,b; Lukas and Griffiths, 1984). The second type involves the study of cross-dependence, in which the animal is made dependent on a compound of known dependence capacity and the ability of the test benzodiazepine to prevent or reverse the withdrawal from the initial compound is examined.

Determination of primary dependence

In this technique the drug is administered regularly to animals over a long period. Under normal circumstances a dose is used which is well above that required to produce pharmacological properties equivalent to that required for human activity. Numerous studies have been undertaken in rats after oral administration of various benzodiazepines (Yanaura *et al.*, 1975; Yanaura and Tagashira, 1975; Nikolova *et al.*, 1975; Yoshimura *et al.*, 1977; Bantutova *et al.*, 1978; Yoshimura and Yamamota, 1979; Ryan and Boisse, 1979; Suzuki *et al.*, 1980; Martin and McNicholas, 1981; Boisse *et al.*, 1978, 1981, 1982).

Other studies have been undertaken in rhesus monkeys and many such studies have been reported from the laboratory directed by Yanagita and summarized in his paper of 1981. Certain qualitative differences have been suggested to occur between the benzodiazepines and barbiturates, but it is far from clear how much these differences are the result of pharmacokinetic considerations rather than the basic effects of the two different classes of drugs.

In most of the studies it has been possible to show withdrawal signs with both rats and rhesus monkeys. In rats, the main effect which has been found has been defined as an 'explosive awakening' (Martin *et al.*, 1982) in which the rat makes a rigid and sudden jump rather than a physical convulsion, although convulsions have been observed. Other withdrawal signs reliably observed after lower doses are weight loss, increased locomotor activity, tremor, muscle rigidity and decreased eating. These mirror the withdrawal effects seen in humans.

Working with rhesus monkeys Yanagita has assigned three different grades to the severity of the withdrawal phenomenon. The first is a mild withdrawal syndrome indicated by apprehension, hyper-irritability, a mild tremor, anorexia and pilo-erection. At the intermediate withdrawal level the tremor becomes more aggravated, rigidity occurs, there is some impairment of motor performance, retching and vomiting and consequent weight loss. During the most severe withdrawal, grand mal convulsions can occur, associated with nystagmus, substantial hyperthermia, dissociation and curious behavioural manifestations.

Most of the studies have been undertaken on large doses of the individual benzodiazepines attempting to obtain very high levels of intoxication. Swain (1983), on the other hand, studying monkeys, used subcutaneous injections, each 6 hours, over a 5 month period with doses that are more in line with those used therapeutically. He studied a 10-day withdrawal

15

period and found that diazepam showed the typical monkey manifestations of withdrawal, suggesting that even at low doses prolonged administration can lead to physical dependence in animal species.

The availability of a benzodiazepine antagonist (Ro 15–1788) has made it possible to abruptly precipitate withdrawal in animals with primary dependence on benzodiazepines. After administration of the antagonist (Haefely *et al.*, 1983) subsequent precipitated withdrawal is believed to result from a direct blockade of the central benzodiazepine receptor.

Based upon the various studies it would appear that all of the benzodiazepines currently available are capable of producing a withdrawal syndrome. There would appear to be some differences between the dose levels at which the grades of withdrawal can occur, but these differences probably depend more on pharmacokinetic considerations than true differences between the dependence liability of the benzodiazepines involved.

Consideration of cross-dependence

In cross-dependence studies a substance is given to the animal until the point when abstinence results in withdrawal phenomena. The test substance is then administered and its ability to suppress the withdrawal phenomena is determined.

The technique is well established for narcotic substances and has been extensively studied in this area. It has also been used for the study of dependence of the sedative alcohol type during which a barbiturate has normally been used to produce the primary dependence. The validity of the concept that cross-substitution implies dependence of a similar type has not been fully tested for the barbiturates and there is a certain amount of doubt whether this concept is valid for this class of dependence. Hence, for example, carisprodol substitutes well for barbital in dogs (Deneau and Weiss, 1968), yet does not appear to produce significant dependence itself (Fraser and Jasinsky, 1977; Fraser *et al.*, 1961).

Thus, all drugs that substitute for a primary compound may not produce the same degree or type of dependence, and theoretically may not produce dependence at all.

Most of the benzodiazepine cross-dependence studies have been undertaken in either rats or mice that have been rendered dependent on either barbital or phenobarbital. Most of the benzodiazepines that have been extensively studied prior to marketing have been subjected to this cross-tolerance test though more studies have been undertaken using chlordiazepoxide or diazepam than on the later compounds in the series. In many of the studies the route of administration, the dose and the time relationship are not adequately described. Nevertheless there is consider-

16

able agreement among the results that have been recorded in such studies (Norton, 1970; Tsuchie *et al.*, 1972; Kaneto *et al.*, 1973; Yanaura *et al.*, 1975; Nikolova *et al.*, 1975; Tagashira *et al.*, 1977; Belknap, 1978; Reigel and Bourn, 1982). These studies show that the various animal withdrawal signs, including audiogenic convulsions, irritability, muscle rigidity and tremor, can be reversed by all the benzodiazepines so far studied.

Other studies have been undertaken in the dog, where barbital withdrawal has been shown to be reversed by benzodiazepines (Deneau and Weiss, 1968; Nikolova *et al.*, 1975). In rhesus monkeys Yanagita and Takahashi (1973) likewise found that diazepam, chlordiazepoxide and oxazepam suppressed signs of barbital withdrawal.

Yanagita (1981) has reviewed the results of the studies undertaken on cross-dependence to barbital in his laboratory (Yanagita *et al.*, 1975a–e, 1977a,b, 1981a–d). These studies showed that all the benzodiazepines examined so far suppressed barbital withdrawal. They differed in potency but there was a high level of correlation between the potency with which the individual benzodiazepine could suppress barbital withdrawal and the affinity constant for the compound to the benzodiazepine receptor as indicated by the displacement of radioactive labelled diazepam (Moehler and Okada, 1977). Certainly there was no indication of an ability to suppress barbital withdrawal that was a function of the benzodiazepines other than that of receptor affinity and pharmacokinetics.

In other experiments alcohol withdrawal has been studied in the rhesus monkey (Miyasato, 1978) and in mice (Blum *et al.*, 1976). Diazepam could reverse alcohol withdrawal in this test, as might be anticipated from the similarity in barbiturate and alcohol dependence phenomena in animals.

SIGNIFICANCE OF THE ANIMAL INVESTIGATIONS

All these results indicate that the benzodiazepines show some activity in experiments involving physical dependence in all species that have been studied. The level of dependence liability in these experiments appears to be significantly less than that of the barbiturates, although the effect is qualitatively similar to that of the barbiturates and alcohol. Any differences that exist may depend more upon pharmacokinetic aspects than on different qualitative or quantitative characteristics of the various benzodiazepines. Hence there is no indication in animal studies that the dependence liability of the members of the benzodiazepine series differs appreciably. Any differences there may be probably relate to pharmacokinetic and receptor binding potency characteristics of these various benzodiazepines.

17

3

Experimental studies on benzodiazepine dependence in humans

Although animal experiments can provide some of the relevant information relating to the development of dependence, it is important to confirm that these results have relevance to the situation in humans, both in terms of therapeutic use and also street abuse.

There are broadly seven different types of experimental study that have been undertaken on the dependence liability of benzodiazepines in the human. The results obtained show differences depending upon the subject group that is studied and the dose used. The overall conclusions from these studies are considered and the ethics of continued work in this area appraised.

EXPERIMENTS THAT DEMONSTRATE THAT DEPENDENCE CAN OCCUR

The classical experiment is that of Hollister and his co-workers (1961). They gave chlordiazepoxide 100–600 mg daily to 36 hospitalized psychotics for periods between 1 and 7 months. Eleven of these patients were abruptly changed to placebo on a single-blind basis and ten of them developed subjective or objective signs interpreted as those of withdrawal (depression in six, aggravation of the psychoses in five, insomnia and agitation in five, anorexia in four, twitching in one and convulsions in three). These symptoms appeared mainly between the 4th and 8th day of withdrawal, corresponding with the half-life data, and were considered to be evidence of dependence.

It is interesting to note that this study has been quoted extensively as evidence for *clinical* dependence on benzodiazepines in normal therapeutic use. Hollister has himself denied (1977) that the work should be

18

regarded in this light since the dose used and the patients treated are not typical of normal therapeutic use. Nevertheless it did indicate that dependence could be produced.

Subsequently Covi *et al.* (1969) showed that when 45 mg/day chlordiazepoxide is administered daily to anxious neurotic patients for either 10 or 20 weeks, abrupt discontinuation produces symptomatic distress (tenseness, trembling, dizziness, anorexia) after the 20 weeks' treatment. They stressed, however, that it is far from clear whether these symptoms were those of withdrawal or of a recurrence of the original anxiety state. This was, however, the first indication that, with doses at the higher end of the therapeutic range and medium length of administration, withdrawal manifestations can occur.

PREFERENCE PARADIGM FOR DIFFERENT SUBJECT POPULATIONS

Normal subjects

The main relevant study in normal subjects is that of Johanson and Uhlenhuth (1980). They examined the preference rating for diazepam (2, 5 or 10 mg) over placebo, for diazepam, (5 mg versus 2 mg), and as a positive control amphetamine (5 mg) over placebo. The subjects were given colour-coded capsules on four occasions and answered questions about mood 1, 3 and 6 hours after each drug administration. Diazepam produced changes in mood that reflected increases in fatigue and confusion and decrease in vigour and arousal. These subjective effects were dose-dependent and most evident 1 hour after the administration. Then after they had experienced each drug or placebo condition twice, the subjects undertook five sessions in which they chose between the capsules while other conditions remained the same. In none of the comparisons was diazepam chosen in more than 50% of the trials. Placebo was chosen more often than either 5 or 10 mg diazepam. On the other hand, amphetamine was preferred significantly over placebo.

Another study carried out in normals was that of DeWit *et al.* (1983), which also looked at the behaviour of anxious patients. The study design was very similar to that used by Johanson and Uhlenhuth (1980) and the test substances were 5 mg diazepam, 10 mg diazepam or 5 mg dl-amphetamine versus placebo. Consistent with the earlier findings of Johanson and Uhlenhuth (1980), the normal subjects did not show a preference for diazepam at either dose. The 5 mg dose was chosen about equally frequently as placebo, but placebo was preferred to the 10 mg dose.

Because the normal volunteers in this experiment were active people, it was thought that the preference for diazepam might be influenced by the time of day, and choice trials were also undertaken in the evening. Amphetamine was preferred less in the evening than in the morning but the diazepam preferences showed no such change, i.e. placebo was preferred to both the 5 and 10 mg dose of diazepam during the day and in the evening.

These studies in normal subjects have been extended by this group using pentobarbital and lorazepam as well as diazepam (de Wit and Johanson, 1983; Johanson and Uhlenhuth, 1982; de Wit et al., 1983, 1984a–c). These studies confirmed the preference for amphetamines over diazepam; lorazepam preference showed the same rating as diazepam with neither showing any preference rating over placebo. Lorazepam showed a longer sedative effect than diazepam despite its shorter half-life; there was no mood elevation with either benzodiazepine; preference for pentobarbital over diazepam and positive mood effects from pentobarbital; no effect of the time of day on these appreciations.

The same group (Chait et al., 1984) have subsequently tried to reinforce drug discrimination by training normal volunteers to discriminate 10 mg d-amphetamine from placebo. Although these trained subjects could subsequently discriminate amphetamine in a dose-dependent fashion, discrimination of diazepam was poor or non-existent.

The Lader group (Bond and Lader, 1981; Lader, 1982; Golombok and Lader, 1984) have also studied drug effects on mood rating using diazepam (5 and 10 mg), prazepam (25 and 50 mg) and buspirone (10 and 20 mg). All these drugs produced drowsiness but no other effects on mood (e.g. contentedness, euphoria).

Anxious patients

Several of these studies have also been undertaken by the Chicago group. The first was that of de Wit et al. (1983) already quoted. A series of subjects were selected who satisfied DSM III for generalized anxiety disorder; subjects with histories of depression or drug abuse were excluded. In this group of anxious patients there was a significant trend towards choosing placebo over 5 mg and 10 mg diazepam. Whereas the normal subjects preferred amphetamine over placebo (those with the amphetamine preference had higher pre-drug anxiety scores (Uhlenhuth et al., 1981), no such preference was seen in the anxious patients (as might be anticipated if depression was excluded).

The subjective effect of the drugs described by the anxious patients was essentially that described by the normal subjects, and they reported a significant reduction in anxiety subsequent to drug ingestion.

In later studies (de Wit et al., 1983, 1984a) the same group could not confirm the preference for diazepam over placebo. There was no preference over placebo at the 5 mg level and they preferred placebo to diazepam 10 mg.

A study by Rickels *et al.* (1977) which examined the clinical effect of halazepam compared with diazepam in neurotic anxiety found that at the end of the study there was a slight patient preference to continue with the benzodiazepine (53% diazepam, 55% halazepam) over placebo (40%).

Other studies that have been undertaken on anxious patients are those reported during the clinical trials of most of the more recently introduced benzodiazepines. As part of the clinical trial, groups of patients who have been receiving the benzodiazepine test compound for periods varying from 3 to 6 months have the substance withdrawn suddenly. None of these reports speak of withdrawal phenomena. However they should be regarded with a certain amount of caution since this was not the prime consideration of the study. Nevertheless it does suggest that for periods up to about 3 to 6 months clinically relevant withdrawal effects are minimal. This aspect will be considered in detail later (Appendix 2).

Insomniacs

There are two preference type studies of benzodiazepines in patients suffering from insomnia, those of Jick *et al.* (1966) and Fabre *et al.* (1976). These show a preference for the benzodiazepine over placebo as measured in the various parameters. However when the benzodiazepine is compared with a barbiturate or with another benzodiazepine, the few preferences that exist depend on the dosage used and pharmacokinetic profiles for each substance. There is no evidence in either of these studies indicating a preference which might lead to higher dependence risk.

Sedative/alcohol abusers

The earliest study was that of Burke and Anderson (1962), who performed an experiment similar to that of Hollister *et al.* (1961) in 25 hospitalized male chronic alcoholics. They were given 75–150 mg/day but for a period of only 2 weeks, but no signs were encountered on sudden withdrawal.

Kryspin-Exner and Demel (1975) assessed the development of tranquillizer dependence in alcoholics supervised in an outpatient setting. They found six (7.7%) among 78 treated with meprobamate, four (3.6%) among 111 treated with chlordiazepoxide and seven (2.3%) among 302 treated with diazepam. Of the 11 who were dependent on the benzodiazepines, seven were already dependent on other medications (e.g. sedatives, analgesics) in addition to the alcohol. They regarded this level of dependence on the benzodiazepines as small in this group with relatively poorly controlled long-term tranquillizer prescription. In a further study with inpatient alcoholics allowed either diazepam (24 patients) or placebo (23 patients) no evidence of diazepam misuse could be found over a 32-day period. The authors then studied a still more difficult group, namely 20 patients who were already dependent on hypnotics (including some with barbiturates). When a combination of oxazepam, diazepam, nitrazepam and lorazepam was administered in an almost unrestricted fashion, eight became dependent, but even this was regarded as less than expected in this population.

Rothstein *et al.* (1976) undertook a study in an outpatient clinic treating patients suffering from alcoholism. Of the 220 patients attending the clinic, 179 were receiving tranquillizers (95% chlordiazepoxide, 4% diazepam and 1% a phenothiazine) to reduce anxiety and tension. Of these, 108 patients were followed up for over a year of tranquillizer medication. The instruction was to use the tranquillizer as necessary for the relief of the symptoms. Eighty-six per cent of the patients did not take the drugs on some days, and 50% omitted them for periods of at least 30 days during the study period. Clinical evidence of dependence was found in only 5% of the group and the authors concluded that even in this group predisposed to abuse, a serious problem was encountered in only 2–3% of the patients.

In two recent studies (Jasinski and Johnson, 1982a,b), the subjective effects of chlordiazepoxide and diazepam have been compared with pentobarbital by volunteer inpatient sedative and alcohol abusers. They reported dose-dependent subjective effects from the benzodiazepines (diazepam 10, 20 and 40 mg) and chlordiazepoxide (100, 200 and 400 mg) similar to those of pentobarbital. The doses used are much higher than those encountered in normal therapeutic practice but are not inappropriate considering the pattern of sedative tolerance found with alcohol and sedative abusers.

Griffiths and his colleagues have also examined the subjective effects of benzodiazepines in similar groups of patients with documented histories of abuse of sedatives and other drugs. In the first study (Griffiths *et al.*, 1976) pentobarbital (30 mg) and diazepam (10 mg) were used as 'rewards' for stationary bicycle riding. The amount of exercise to produce a reward was varied and the response to each drug was reduced as the exercise level was increased. Both drugs maintained self-administration, however, throughout the test.

In the second study (Griffiths *et al.*, (1979) male volunteers were given an opportunity on the first day to become familiar with the drug to be used as reinforcer by being able to request up to 10 doses at intervals of at least 15 minutes between doses. Then over the succeeding 10-day test period, the volunteers were required to ride a stationary bicycle for 15 minutes in order to receive a drug 'reward'. Neither dose of chlorpromazine (25 or 50 mg) was distinguished from placebo. Pentobarbital (30 mg) maintained two to four ingestions per day towards the end of the period, while 90 mg maintained six to nine ingestions rather regularly over the whole period. Diazepam 20 mg produced more response than 10 mg but both declined over the 10-day period and if continued would probably not have produced a response rate greater than placebo. The staff- and self-rating of the subjective effects suggested that the subjective effects of the higher doses of pentobarbital and diazepam were equivalent but the barbiturate produced more consistent self-administration than the benzodiazepine.

Later studies by the Griffiths group (Griffiths *et al.*, 1983; Funderburke *et al.*, 1983; Griffiths *et al.*, 1984) have confirmed a dose-dependent preference for diazepam (40, 80 and 160 mg) over placebo in the sedative abuse group. The maximum diazepam effect was seen at 1–2 hours compared with the 8–12 hours for oxazepam. In their studies 60 mg of diazepam could be equated by extrapolation with 480 mg oxazepam on preference rating. The relaxation effect of diazepam and its rapid onset of action were cited as positive aspects. Diazepam doses of 10, 20 and 40 mg corresponded to lorazepam 1.5, 3 and 6 mg on the preference scale, though the lorazepam effect was longer-lasting despite its more rapid elimination.

Cole *et al.* (1982a) compared diazepam 10 and 20 mg with buspirone 40 mg and placebo on the ARC I stimulation–euphoria scale in recreational drug abusers and found that diazepam was more euphoriant than either buspirone or placebo but that the effect was small. In a further study (Cole *et al.*, 1982b,c), diazepam (10 mg) appeared to be slightly more euphoriant than prazepam (20 mg) but less so than methaqualone (200 and 400 mg).

The study by Jaffe *et al.* (1983) was carried out on 30 men who had just completed alcohol withdrawal. They compared the euphoric and drug-liking effects of halazepam (160 and 320 mg) diazepam (20 and 40 mg) and placebo. At 30 minutes the diazepam group already showed a euphoriant effect while the halazepam group showed no subjective effects. By 2–3 hours halazepam at both doses showed some subjective effects but less than the peak effects for diazepam. While this study suggests a greater euphoriant effect for diazepam than halazepam, there are doubts about the relevance and validity of the study (e.g. single doses; post-withdrawal alcoholics (i.e. any liver dysfunction would delay halazepam conversion to the active form); no dose-dependence in halazepam; *post hoc* re-evaluation of data before analysis).

Abusers of multiple drugs

It is not always easy to distinguish these studies on drug abusers of multiple drugs from those of sedatives and alcohol because the reports are not always clear on the totality of the drugs that are being abused by the volunteers. Hence these studies should also be considered together with those recorded in the previous section.

Griffiths *et al.* (1976) studied the self-administration of pentobarbital, diazepam or ethanol in a ward situation on volunteers with fully documented evidence of multiple drug abuse. The total of each substance taken varied with the dose and time interval but the overall pattern was similar for each of the three drugs, suggesting that the dependence liability was broadly similar for each.

In a later study Griffiths *et al.* (1980) studied the drug and dose preference using a variety of doses of pentobarbital (200–900 mg) and diazepam (50–400 mg) compared with placebo in a similar group. It is clear that the doses used were far in excess of those in the previous experiments and well above those encountered in therapeutic practice. Increasing the dose of pentobarbital led to increases in the subjective reports of drug effect and to increase in preference. On the other hand in the diazepam study there were only minimal subjective effects up to the 400 mg and no marked preference for the higher dose. When pentobarbital (400 mg) and diazepam (200 mg) were compared under comparable conditions each subject expressed a preference for pentobarbital, though the diazepam was preferred over placebo, despite the limited subjective effects experienced.

In recent studies, the Griffiths group (Roache and Griffiths 1983, 1984) attempted to define the abuse liability of diazepam 10–160 mg; oxazepam 30–480 mg; triazolam 0.5–3.0 mg and pentobarbital 100–600 mg by various objective and subjective measurements. These studies have only been published to date in abstract form. The abstracts suggest that though there are differences in detailed aspects of drug-liking (peak effect and time course) these are probably related to pharmacokinetic aspects.

Healey and Pickens (1983) studied drug preference to diazepam (2–40 mg) or pentobarbital (30 or 50 mg) in a double-blind preference experiment over 24-hour periods in 10 subjects with drug-abuse histories. When diazepam 5 or 10 mg was used as the standard, there was no dose preference among any of the diazepam doses. With 30 or 50 mg pentobarbital as the standard, there was consistent dose-dependent diazepam preference among three of the four male subjects, whereas in the six females no consistent diazepam dose preference was observed. There were no obvious reasons for these differences.

Psychiatric patients

Winstead *et al.* (1974) assessed a number of features of diazepam in a 16-bed general psychiatric ward setting over a period of 6 months. Other medications were prescribed as necessary but diazepam (10 mg doses) could be requested from the staff at any time. They reported a positive relation between the anxiety level and the diazepam requests and the number of requests declined over the 6-month period from an average of one request per 2 days to one request every 4 days.

A study of a rather similar type to that of Winstead *et al.* (1974) was also reported by Balmer *et al.* (1981). This involved 54 outpatients with neurotic disorders who were instructed to use up to six tablets of diazepam (5 mg) or placebo daily, the drug supply being replaced as necessary. Over the course of the 6-month study use of both the placebo and the diazepam declined, with a more rapid decline of the placebo. High diazepam intake was related to severe anxiety symptoms but no similar correlation was present for the placebo. Over the period of the study slightly over one diazepam and slightly less than one placebo tablet was consumed daily per patient on average.

Both these studies, which are supported by several observations of drug self-administration in psychiatric settings, indicate that when a benzodiazepine is available on demand there is no evidence of high intake (see also p. 72) and the level of intake follows very closely the level of anxiety and tends to decline with time.

APPRAISAL OF THE HUMAN EXPERIMENTAL STUDIES

These experiments in humans confirm and extend those undertaken in animals. The benzodiazepines that have been studied carefully (mainly the earlier and more widely used preparations – particularly diazepam) will produce a reinforcing effect in doses that are only slightly above the therapeutic range in humans (normals or those suffering from a psychiatric disorder). The level of reinforcement is low and certainly less than that of barbiturates with an equivalent sedative effect. In normal subjects and those who use the drugs therapeutically it is very difficult to determine a preference effect that cannot be explained purely on the basis of the therapeutic activity. In sedative abusers, on the other hand, larger doses of benzodiazepines (diazepam (20–200 mg) is the drug that has mainly been studied) may support a preference but this is not consistent and since the techniques used are different this may only represent procedural differences. There are considerable difficulties over the interpretation of the observations due to different pharmacokinetic profiles; including both speed and duration of action and time to maximum effect.

Certainly no human experimental study indicates a substantial drive for use or abuse of a benzodiazepine and, in fact, voluntary benzodiazepine consumption generally declines over time. In this respect it is interesting to note that benzodiazepine abuse does not show the 'career pathway' leading to the abuse of other drugs such as occurs with cannabis

(Kandel and Logan, 1984; Yamaguchi and Kandel, 1984a,b) or solvent abusers (Davies *et al.*, 1985).

ETHICAL CONSIDERATIONS

Since it is now known that benzodiazepines can produce both physical and psychological dependence, and that in extreme cases the withdrawal manifestations can include both convulsions and psychotic reactions, the ethical aspects of further human experimental studies require consideration.

It is abundantly clear that such studies can only be undertaken if the volunteer or patient has been fully informed about the unpleasant nature of the withdrawal effects and the risks involved, and gives permission of their own freewill, knowing all the facts. With a clear indication that dependence can be produced, there would seem to be grave doubts about the ethics of studies on normals, or long-term studies on those with anxiety or insomnia. On the other hand studies on known abusers of drugs are of very doubtful validity relative to the population at therapeutic risk.

It is also clear now (p. 76) that even when dependence is present, the severity of the withdrawal manifestations can be considerably reduced by gradual withdrawal and there would therefore appear to be considerable doubt about the ethics of studies that require sudden withdrawal as part of their protocol, in order to produce observable signs of dependence.

It would therefore seem that unless the investigation forms part of a genuine treatment regime that can be fully justified in its own right, studies must now be restricted to those that are of short-term duration (probably not more than 2 weeks ideally) and even then do not involve sudden withdrawal. This probably largely restricts them to preference trials. This must be regarded as an unfortunate restriction in view of the amount of further information that is still required, but is nevertheless ethically important.

4
Patterns of benzodiazepine dependence

On the basis of personal experience and appraisal of the literature the author has reached the conclusion that there is not one single entity of benzodiazepine dependence but a collection of disorders which show sufficient differences to be regarded as separate, though related, phenomena (see also Ayd, 1981, who expresses similar views).

BENZODIAZEPINE PHYSICAL AND PSYCHOLOGICAL DEPENDENCE DURING THERAPEUTIC USE

The long-term therapeutic daily ingestion of benzodiazepines carries with it a substantial risk of both physical and psychological dependence. The time interval below which dependence is very rare, and the ultimate proportion of the population at risk that became dependent, are matters of dispute and are considered in detail in other parts of the book (Appendix 2).

The incidence of dependence during therapeutic use is probably greater in those with a 'dependence liability' or with neurotic disorders, but a risk exists within those who are treated for physical ills – e.g. spastic disorders. The important and unusual feature which distinguishes the majority of this therapeutically induced benzodiazepine dependence from that which occurs as a result of the administration of other sedatives is that, with the benzodiazepines, the daily dosage is either unaltered or minimally increased. Some degree of tolerance can be demonstrated by experimental procedures (Peturrson and Lader, 1984), but tolerance is not normally a clinical problem.

Hence this type of benzodiazepine dependence does not show all the classical features of substance dependence according to WHO criteria (i.e. there is no clear tolerance). This feature of normal dosage also makes it more difficult to distinguish those who maintain therapy to avoid

27

abstinence phenomena from those who require long-term therapy to treat chronic anxiety.

While it is clear that the encouragement of dependence by inappropriate therapy should be avoided, it is suggested that the current actual level of dependence as a result of therapeutic use generates a greater level of emotion, particularly among lay people, than is justified by medical considerations. This is commented on in greater detail elsewhere (p. 72 *et seq.*). Specifically we agree with those who contend that inappropriate lay publicity has resulted in patients experiencing the abstinence syndrome who would not otherwise have done so (Winokur and Rickels, 1981) and also led to patients not receiving adequate anti-anxiety relief.

BENZODIAZEPINE ABUSER GROUP

There is a small group of people who only abuse one benzodiazepine, but do so at substantial dosage. It appears that the majority of these people originally started to use the benzodiazepine in the therapeutic milieu, then as a result of tolerance which, as explained above, is unusual, steadily increased their dosage until the daily intake may be 20–50 times the therapeutic dose. Despite the high dose they show minimal sedation.

It is interesting to note that this type of patient is seldom encountered in the United States (Ayd, 1981), the United Kingdom, most of Europe and many other parts of the world. However, there are extensive reports of this type of patient in Germany over the past 5 years (Kemper *et al.*, 1980; Hippius and Ruther, 1982; van Oefele *et al.*, 1983; Binder *et al.*, 1984). The reason for this local problem is unknown.

Benzodiazepine dependence in the sedative abuser group

A substantial group of people exists who abuse sedative drugs, usually consuming both alcohol and an hypnotic during each 24 hour period. They should be distinguished from the alcoholic, who occasionally takes a sleeping pill, by the regularity of the utilization of both alcohol *and* the sedative. Such people have in the past been heavy users of barbiturates, but recently with the reduced availability of the barbiturates and increased ease of acquiring benzodiazepines, these latter substances are being substituted. If sedative abuse cannot be totally avoided the substitution should be welcomed, for the combination of barbiturates and alcohol is more likely to be lethal than a benzodiazepine and alcohol. However, as Lader (1980b) has pointed out, such people prefer barbiturates and alcohol if they are available.

BENZODIAZEPINE DEPENDENCE IN THE STREET SCENE: MULTIPLE DRUG ABUSE

The fourth, separate group of benzodiazepine dependence subjects are those who use it within the street drug abuse scene. This group is considered in more detail in Chapter 8. They abuse hard drugs and add to this other substances either to reduce the unpleasant features of their prime abuse, to increase the degree of intoxication or to cushion withdrawal symptoms when there are supply problems for hard drugs.

It is important to appreciate that benzodiazepine abuse does not lead on to hard drug abuse though the reverse does occur. However, as Ayd (1981) stresses, the benzodiazepine is added to the hard drug. There is no known case of a street drug abuser 'abandoning hard drugs in favour of diazepam' or any benzodiazepine. The hard drugs involved are usually narcotics and it is far less usual to find benzodiazepine abuse among cocaine takers (Budd, 1981).

5
The pathophysiological mechanisms of benzodiazepine dependence

The discovery of high-affinity binding sites for benzodiazepines through-out the central nervous system in 1977 (Braestrup and Squires, 1977; Moehler and Okada, 1977; Squires and Braestrup, 1977) opened up the possibility for explaining the action of benzodiazepines at cellular level.

The affinity of benzodiazepines for the binding sites correlated well with their pharmacological and clinical potency, providing evidence that they might represent true drug receptors for benzodiazepines. It had previously been suggested that benzodiazepines enhanced GABA-ergic transmission (Haefely *et al.*, 1975; Costa *et al.*, 1975) and it is currently suggested that benzodiazepine binding sites form one component of a supramolecular complex which also contains the GABA receptor and chloride channel. Barbiturates and picrotoxin can attach to other parts of the complex. GABA-mediated changes in chloride movements could lead to changes in the level of inhibition in the central nervous system. A hypothetical model of the current view of the benzodiazepine–GABA–chloride channel is shown in Figure 2, based on one of the recent reviews on the synaptic mechanism (Haefely *et al.*, 1983).

Natural ligands for the receptor are postulated, which would either be the natural anxiolytic–sedative components that maintain psychological normality; or anxiety-provoking natural substances that act as antagon-ists somewhere on the receptor complex.

Against this background it is scarcely surprising that receptor changes or interactions have been held to play a role in the development of dependence and tolerance. Several investigations have been aimed at demonstrating alterations of affinity or density of the binding sites in association with the development of tolerance. So far there is no convinc-ing evidence of changes in these sites occurring with prolonged adminis-tration of benzodiazepines (Haefely *et al.*, 1983).

30

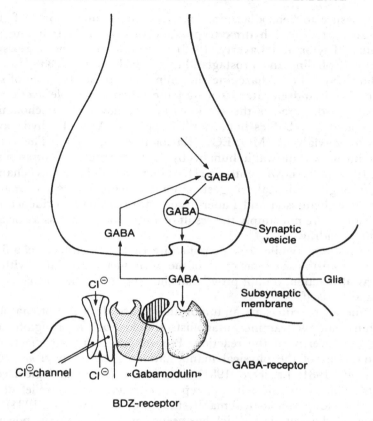

Figure 2 A representation of the chloride channel and the factors that affect it (based on Haefely *et al.*, 1983)

The development of withdrawal symptoms is related to the rate at which blood (and by analogy tissue) levels of the benzodiazepines fall. Those benzodiazepines that persist in the body show a delayed onset of abstinence phenomena. On the other hand rapidly eliminated representatives of the series provoke florid withdrawal effects more rapidly after the drugs are stopped. Moreover the administration of an antagonist to the benzodiazepine receptor (Ro 15–1788), leads to a dramatic withdrawal phenomenon, at least in the animal model.

Hence the current concept of the withdrawal phenomenon is based upon either a rebound hypersensitivity of the receptor or loss of the unnatural ligand (the benzodiazepine) before regeneration of the natural ligand.

The GABA-ergic neurons involved are known to be inhibitory to various amine-mediated central synaptic activities. Thus acute or subacute exposure to benzodiazepines reduces the brain turnover of such neurotransmitters as 5-hydroxytryptamine (5-HT), noradrenaline and dopamine (Taylor and Laverty, 1969) as well as neuromodulators including enkephalins and prostaglandins (Haefely et al., 1983).

Withdrawal of benzodiazepines in animals decreases the rate of synthesis of 5-HT and elevates its metabolite 5-hydroxyindole acetic acid (5-HIAA), and increases the synthesis and turnover of catecholamine with elevated metabolites homovanillic acid (HVA) and 4-hydroxy-3-methoxy-phenylglycol (MOPEG) (Rastogni et al., 1978). The recent studies during withdrawal in humans by the Lader group (Petursson and Lader, 1984) have shown similar 5-HIAA increases and MOPEG changes which, though equivocal, suggest a human neurochemical change of similar type. Petursson and Lader argue with reasonable evidence that these changes are not simply the result of a non-specific stress associated with the withdrawal.

These findings, while they demonstrate that aminergic mechanisms may be responsible for some or all of the phenomena associated with the withdrawal reaction, do not prove that they represent the mechanism of the reaction itself.

If aminergic reactions are an important feature of the symptomatology of withdrawal, then amine antagonists should abolish or significantly reduce the severity of the reaction. Propranolol is indeed effective in reducing some of the physical manifestations (Abernethy et al., 1981; Tyrer et al., 1981; Lapierre, 1981) though not the psychological components. This is in line with its reported activity in the relief of the somatic but not psychological manifestations of anxiety (Peet, 1984). On the other hand oxypertine, which has been thought to be a more powerful adrenergic inhibitor, is ineffective in the relief of either the somatic or psychological manifestations (Peturrson and Lader, 1984).

Hence though there is a priori evidence that benzodiazepine dependence and abstinence syndrome are dependent on changes in the specific receptor, and that at least some of the peripheral effects are aminergic-dependent (possible 5-HT) there are still vast gaps in our knowledge of the cellular mechanisms that are involved.

At the behavioural level Gray et al. (1983) postulated the existence of a 'behavioural inhibition system' within part of the limbic system. This is an area known to be rich in GABA, with a high density of benzodiazepine-specific receptor sites and, on the basis of electropharmacological studies, to be sensitive to benzodiazepines. According to the Gray hypothesis this system responds to anxiety-provoking stimuli, increasing arousal and attention but producing behavioural inhibition. On this basis the drug dependence-producing properties exerted by benzodiazepines and other sedatives could be explained by amnesic inhibition of a state-dependent learning involving that system (Jensen and Poulsen, 1982).

32

6
Description of the benzodiazepine withdrawal reaction

CLINICAL

Physical dependence

The clinical manifestations of a benzodiazepine abstinence syndrome, implying physical dependence, resemble those that occur with sedatives, including barbiturates, and with alcohol, but show some difference of time and degree rather than nature. Among the most extensive studies describing the withdrawal clinical disorder are those of Tyrer *et al.* (1981), Smith and Wesson (1983) and Petursson and Lader (1984).

Since the half-lives of many of the widely used benzodiazepines are substantially longer than those of the majority of sedatives, the fall in the blood levels is more gradual, and levels low enough to precipitate the abstinence syndrome occur later after withdrawal of the drug – usually on the third to the sixth day. Moreover the symptoms and signs may last for a shorter time and be less florid than those seen with other sedatives.

For those benzodiazepines that are rapidly eliminated from the body (e.g. lorazepan) the withdrawal reaction occurs earlier and, due to the rapid fall in the plasma level, tends to be more florid. Whether with the ultra- short-acting benzodiazepines with a half-life below about 5 hours, a withdrawal reaction will occur after each dose in those who use the substances at higher doses for a prolonged period, is a matter of current dispute. Some (Morgan and Oswald, 1982; Kales *et al.*, 1979) have suggested that this is a common feature with the short-acting drugs but this has been denied by, for example, Nicholson *et al.* (1982). Hollister (1977), based on experience with other sedatives (mainly barbiturates), has suggested that there is a maximum severity of withdrawal manifestations at a half-life of about 12-15 hours and that sedatives with a

33

substantially shorter or longer half-life will show less florid withdrawal effects. The evidence on this for the benzodiazepines is equivocal.

In its most minor form, patients during withdrawal will suffer little more than anxiety, apprehension, insomnia, dizziness and anorexia, and these manifestations occurred in virtually every one of the selected group of patients studied by Petursson and Lader (1984).

The manifestations of moderate degrees of withdrawal are those already described for minor cases together with a large number of other symptoms and signs (Hollister *et al.*, 1961; Barten, 1965; Darcy, 1972; Nerenz, 1974; Fruensgaard and Vaag, 1975; Vyas and Carney, 1975; Fruensgaard, 1976; Floyd and Murphy, 1976; Rifkin *et al.*, 1976; Dysken and Chan, 1977; Preskorn and Denner, 1977; Allgulander and Borg, 1978; Acuda and Muhangi, 1979; de Bard, 1979; Bismuth *et al.*, 1980; de la Fuente *et al.*, 1980; Einarson, 1980; Howe, 1980; Kemper *et al.*, 1980; Khan *et al.*, 1980; Le Bellec *et al.*, 1980; Hallstrom and Lader, 1981; Tyrer *et al.*, 1981; Haslerud and Heskestad, 1981; Petursson and Lader, 1981b). These can be categorized as:

(a) *Psychological manifestations* of anxiety – including irritability, increased anxiety and tension, agitation, restlessness, difficulty in concentration, feelings of foreboding, panic attacks.

(b) *Physiological correlates of anxiety* – including tremor, shakiness, headache, profuse sweating, palpitations, insomnia.

(c) *Hyperexcitability and perceptual changes of hyperacuity* – including muscle twitching, muscle aches and pains, hyperacuity to light, sound, touch, pain and smell, a metallic taste.

(d) *Other physical disorders* – including nausea, retching, loss of appetite, weight loss, 'flu-like' illness.

(e) *Other psychological reactions* – including dysphoria, impaired memory, depersonalization and derealization, psychotic reactions, hallucinations, paranoid ideation and depressions.

Of these the psychological and physiological manifestations of anxiety are found in the majority of patients, hyperacuity and other physical disturbances are present in about half the patients and other psychological reactions are found in under 25% of withdrawal reactions (Petursson and Lader, 1981b, 1984).

In its most severe form the benzodiazepine abstinence syndrome adds to the manifestations already described: seizures: (Hollister *et al.*, 1961; Barten, 1965; Nerenz, 1974; Vyas and Carney, 1975; Fruensgaard, 1976; Rifkin *et al.*, 1976; Acuda and Muhangi, 1979; de Bard, 1979; Bismuth *et al.*, 1980; de la Fuente *et al.*, 1980; Einarson, 1980; Howe, 1980; Kemper *et al.*, 1980; Khan *et al.*, 1980; Le Bellec *et al.*, 1980; Hallstrom and Lader, 1981; Tyrer *et al.*, 1981); marked psychotic reactions (Hollister *et al.*, 1961; Barten, 1965; Darcy, 1972; Fruensgaard and Vaag, 1975; Floyd and Murphy, 1976; Fruensgaard, 1976; Dysken and Chan, 1977; Preskorn and Denner, 1977; Allgulander and Borg, 1978; de Bard, 1979; Bismuth *et al.*, 1980; Kemper *et al.*, 1980; Hallstrom and Lader, 1981; Haslerud and Heskestad, 1981; Petursson and Lader, 1981). Hyperthermia and exhaustion leading to a fatal outcome (Relkin, 1966) may also occur, though such severity is excessively rare with the benzodiazepines.

There are difficulties in determining with certainty in the individual patient if the less florid manifestations really represent physical dependence for the following reasons:

(a) Rebound: rebound reactions are very common with many drugs, the majority of which are not implicated in dependence (Lupolover *et al.*, 1982). Several of the objective signs related to benzodiazepine withdrawal can be shown to be due to rebound (Petursson and Lader, 1984), and can occur after short-term, high-dose therapy when there is no implication or evidence of dependence. Some of the anxiety phenomena and insomnia found after the benzodiazepine is stopped probably fall into this category.

(b) Non-specific symptomatology: as Merz (Merz, 1982; Merz and Ballmer, 1983) has shown, about one in ten of the normal population, and a higher proportion of those typically prescribed tranquillizers, present a substantial proportion (between one-third and two-thirds) of the list of symptoms that are quoted in withdrawal reaction papers. Hence a substantial proportion of the symptoms may represent the usual feelings of both normal and, more especially, anxious subjects.

(c) Recurrence of anxiety: Rickels (1982) has stressed that anxiety, the main disorder for which the benzodiazepines are prescribed, is typically a recurrent disorder. Too short a period of treatment, Rickels points out, leads to a higher risk of recurrence. On the other hand it is abundantly clear that a proportion of patients have become dependent as a direct result of the physician reinstituting therapy on frequent occasions in the belief (probably correct initially) that they were treating a recurrent and uncured anxiety state.

Differential diagnosis of withdrawal reactions

The distinction between the two disorders (i.e. return of the anxiety and withdrawal phenomenon) is among the most difficult in medicine. Many authors (e.g. Hollister (1980); Rickels (1981); Smith and Wesson (1983)), have stressed the differential diagnostic importance of the time sequence of the two disorders.

According to these views, with a long-acting benzodiazepine the withdrawal phenomenon starts approximately 2–3 days after the drug is withdrawn, reaches a maximum at about 7–8 days, and then reduces in intensity. On the other hand the return of an anxiety state comes on rather more slowly and gradually reaches the higher level about 2–3 weeks after the drug is withdrawn and persists at this level (Figure 3).

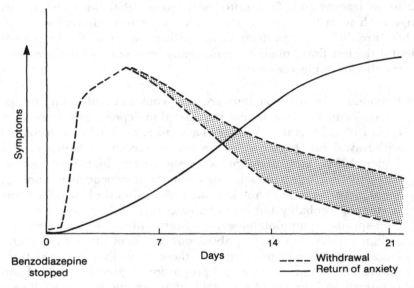

Figure 3 The time sequence for the symptoms of withdrawal from long-acting benzodiazepines contrasted with the typical return of an inadequately treated anxiety

The author has seen several patients with a withdrawal reaction from the medium to long half-life benzodiazepines who have followed the typical pattern and this is also the picture described by those who have worked extensively in the field. However, there have been various reports of prolonged reactions after withdrawal (Schopf, 1981; Oswald and Priest, 1965; Ayd, 1983). Petursson and Lader (1984) also stress that the depressive reaction occurred 2–4 weeks after withdrawal. This report of the studies of the Lader group also demonstrates that many of the post-withdrawal abnormalities have not returned to normal by day 49 or even at follow-up 3 months after completion of the withdrawal period.

This second phase withdrawal reaction with a maximum intensity after 3 weeks was also reported by Mellor and Jain (1982), who drew attention to the fact that many of these later symptoms were the result of hyperacuity. This would also accord with the views of Trickett (1984) that many patients have a prolonged period of poor health after withdrawal. Most of the evidence produced by Trickett is anecdotal and takes no cognizance of the incidence of intercurrent illnesses nor of the personality of the individual. Nevertheless the incidence of prolonged disturbance to health is such that considerable caution should be exercised by doctors in the post-withdrawal follow-up period lest they treat by drugs an iatrogenic disorder and perpetuate the problem. The whole question of the duration of the withdrawal reaction would appear to need further study.

The other aspect which helps to distinguish between the withdrawal reaction and a return of a recurrent anxiety is the presence of certain bizarre symptomatology in the withdrawal reactions, and specifically several that are only seen very rarely in situational anxiety states. These include depersonalization and derealization, and the hyperacuity symptomatology of increased awareness of colour, form, smell and taste.

Precipitation of convulsions

One method of dealing with the abstinence syndrome that has been widely advocated is the administration of antipsychotic drugs in low dosage (particularly phenothiazines). Alternatively the doctor may decide that the patient is depressed, withdraw the benzodiazepine and substitute a tricyclic antidepressant. *Each of these procedures should, in my opinion, be avoided* for each may be dangerous. It is known that phenothiazines and the related tricyclic antidepressants (Peck *et al.*, 1983; Edwards and Glenn-Bott, 1984) lower the convulsive threshold and from the literature survey it appears that a disproportionately high number of those who have developed convulsions upon withdrawal had received antipsychotic or antidepressant therapy during the withdrawal period. This phenomenon has also been noted by Smith (1979); Mellerio (1980); Lapierre (1981); Bismuth *et al.*, (1981); Hartviksen (1981); Haslerud and Heskestad (1981); Barton (1981); Robinson and Sellers (1982); Edwards and Glen-Bott (1984).

Psychological dependence

While many of those working in the field of drug dependence suggest that psychological dependence is a constant accompaniment of physical dependence, it is often difficult to confirm its existence for the benzodiazepines. The essential feature of psychological dependence is the drug-seeking compulsion and, since the benzodiazepines do not usually show tolerance and are so widely available on prescription, the drug-seeking behaviour is not so obvious.

In those unusual cases in which tolerance is a feature, the drive to obtain tablets increases, tolerance is likely, the patient returns before the previous supply of tablets merits it, demands rather than requests larger supplies, and may be found to be attending two different physicians to obtain the drug. Once it reaches this florid state psychological dependence is obvious. At the more usual levels with the benzodiazepines diagnosis will be difficult.

37

PSYCHOPATHOLOGY

The Lader group (Lader *et al.*, 1980; Petursson and Lader, 1981; Hallstrom and Lader, 1981; Petursson and Lader, 1984) have studied various psychophysiological and psychological parameters during the withdrawal phase. The electroencephalogram showed a marked drop in fast-wave activity and an increase in activity in the slower frequency areas; an increase in the auditory-evoked EEG responses. There is an increase in the mean skin conductance. All these responses showed time–response curves of a type similar to that seen after barbiturate withdrawal. Whether the changes were indicative of rebound hyperexcitability and arousal akin to the clinical hyperacuity is far from clear.

They also tested the reaction time, the digit symbol substitution test, symbol copying test, cancellation task, decision time and key tapping test. Unfortunately, as the authors admit, interpretation of these studies is difficult because of substantial learning effects coupled with inadequate controls.

BIOCHEMICAL PATHOLOGY

The same investigators (Petursson and Lader, 1984) have also undertaken biochemical assays during the withdrawal phase. They investigated the two conjugates of 4-hydroxy-3-methoxy-phenylglycol (MOPEG), the 5-hydroxy-indole acetic acid level (5-HIAA) and the 3-methoxy-4-hydroxy-mandelic acid (HMMA) levels in the urine.

MOPEG excretion was greatly reduced during the phase of chronic treatment and levels increased upon discontinuation of the benzodiazepine. The concentration of MOPEG was always less than that of controls during the post-withdrawal phase. This probably reflected the greater urine volumes in the patient group, since the excretion expressed per gram of creatinine did not differ significantly from the control values 3 weeks after withdrawal. The HMMA values were all within the normal range. 5-HIAA values increased during benzodiazepine withdrawal, reached a maximum about 2 weeks after withdrawal and then declined.

Cortisol values showed no significant changes during the period.

The curve for 5-HIAA coupled with that for MOPEG is consistent with the changes in amine levels which would mirror the observed neurological stress reaction. They probably represent peripheral changes, with possibly some alterations within the nervous system. However the stress must be of non-specific type since there was no increase in the cortisol level.

7
Literature appraisal – Benzodiazepine dependence during therapeutic use

Since the initial human experiments conducted by Hollister *et al.* in 1961, it has been clear that the benzodiazepines (like most psychotropic drugs) if given in large enough doses for a long enough period could lead to physical and psychological dependence in most if not all subjects.

Following a review of the world literature a few years ago, I concluded that the benzodiazepines, specifically the 1,4-benzodiazepines had a negligible dependence risk as used in therapy (Marks, 1978). However recent published evidence suggests that a reappraisal is desirable.

The benzodiazepines were originally used by, or under the immediate direction of, psychiatrists. Now the majority of use is by general practitioners, and psychiatrists mainly see the therapeutic failures. In consequence new problems have emerged.

LITERATURE UPDATE

In the 1978 monograph I surveyed the world literature from the introduction of the benzodiazepines in 1960 to mid-1977: 118 papers reported 458 patients in whom there was *a priori* evidence of benzodiazepine dependence, although the evidence was in many cases slender (Marks, 1978). By the end of 1984* the number of publications with individual cases reported had risen to 199 with a total of 848 patients, details of whom are recorded in Appendix 1. It is this current situation to 1984 that is reviewed here.

In addition to these papers which report individual patients, either in

* The final literature search was undertaken during January 1985. It is believed to be accurate to July 1984 for all languages and also covers English-language papers in major journals for most of 1984.

39

detail or in such a way that they can be identified, there are now several reports covering major series (Allgulander, 1978; Kemper *et al.*, 1980; Smith and Wesson, 1983; Busto *et al.*, 1983b; Van Oefele *et al.*, 1983; Binder *et al.*, 1984). These cover some 700 additional cases, many in the socio-recreational abuse situation and often with other drugs. Since it is not possible to analyse these acurately they have not been included in Appendix 1.

From the early papers it has been apparent that published cases have occurred under three distinct circumstances: 'socio-recreational abuse', effect on the fetus of use in mother, and as a result of therapeutic use.

ABUSE

From the early analysis of the total reported cases it was clear that the majority occur in circumstances of abuse, usually with alcohol or other drugs. In this respect it is interesting to note that it is the exception for any of the benzodiazepines to be a drug of primary abuse. Rarely, pure abuse of very high doses of benzodiazepines is reported.

As Smith (Smith and Wesson, 1983; Smith and Marks, 1985) has stressed, narcotics are drugs of primary dependence but benzodiazepines not; the latter are used mainly to reduce the side-effects. The question of benzodiazepine abuse in the socio-recreational situation is considered in detail in Chapter 8. This present chapter is concerned with dependence under therapeutic circumstances in neonates or patients.

WITHDRAWAL REACTIONS IN NEONATES

These have been reported following administration of benzodiazepines to the mothers during the later stages of pregnancy (Bitnum, 1969; Athmarayanan *et al.*, 1976; Mazzi, 1977; Rementeria and Bhatt, 1977; Rane *et al.*, 1979; Backes and Cordero, 1980). The majority of the cases reported to date have resulted from the administration of long-acting benzodiazepines, and the manifestations have appeared between a few hours and few days after delivery, depending on how long before delivery the benzodiazepine was discontinued. At the least there may be tremor, irritability, high-pitched cry and poor feeding. At the worst EEG changes may be present. No case of neonatal fits has been reported yet, but the rare case would appear possible in theory. The withdrawal disorder should be distinguished from the 'floppy baby' syndrome produced by many sedatives given to the mother about the onset of delivery (Gillberg, 1977).

DEPENDENCE DURING THERAPEUTIC USE

A significant change from the 1978 analysis has been the incidence of clear evidence of a withdrawal reaction when normal therapeutic doses have been suddenly withdrawn from patients not known to be dependent on, or currently using, either alcohol or cross-reacting sedatives or hypnotics. In order to examine these features of dependence more carefully I have analysed the data on 188 patients in whom details of the dosage levels, length of administration, etc., are recorded. Cases of multiple benzodiazepine use were excluded.

Age and sex

The age was recorded for 263 patients. The average age was 39 years with a distribution shown in Figure 4, in which it is compared with the distribution of ages recorded in the 1979 survey of use in the United States by Mellinger and Balter (1981). Age distribution of use similar to that found by Mellinger and Balter (1981) has been reported in a 1977 survey in England by Murray *et al.* (1981).

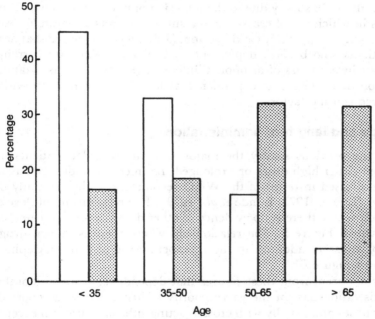

Figure 4 A comparison of the age of the withdrawal cases (open columns) (based on those in Appendix 1 capable of analysis) with the age of users (shaded) (based on Mellinger and Balter, 1981)

The sex was recorded in 315 patients. The number of men (160) and women (155) was almost equal. This contrasts with the ratio of about 2 women to 1 man found in all tranquillizer *user* surveys over the past several years.

Thus it is clear that the published cases of dependence are not typical of the whole population at risk. On the evidence available it is not possible to explain why there is a younger age group with a higher proportion of males. It cannot represent socio-recreational cases since these have been excluded. It would appear unlikely that the difference would have resulted from more rigorous reporting of younger male cases. On the other hand it is possible that older female patients are less willing to be withdrawn from medication, and hence do not demonstrate withdrawal phenomena. Another possible explanation is the predisposing effect of simultaneous ingestion of alcohol (Smith and Wesson, 1983) which is used more frequently by men.

Misuse of other drugs

The high proportion of patients who had previously been or still were recorded consumers of alcohol or sedative hypnotic drugs noted in the previous survey was confirmed. The percentage is, however, now less than in the 1978 survey due to the inclusion of patients from withdrawal studies in which use of cross-reacting substances was a reason for exclusion from the study. Smith and Wesson, (1983) have suggested that nearly all patients who become dependent on benzodiazepines are current or previous heavy users of alcohol. While we agree that the association is common, it is clear that dependence at low dosage can occur without this predisposing factor.

Dosage and length of administration

As in the previous survey the majority of the recorded patients have received either high doses or prolonged treatment. The dosage has now been expressed in terms of the WHO recommended defined daily dose (DDD) (Lunde, 1977; Lunde *et al.*, 1979). The relationship of dose and duration where there is no evidence of other drugs or alcohol being used is shown in Figure 5. The relationship where there is known drug or alcohol abuse in addition to the therapeutic use of benzodiazepines is shown in Figure 6.

It is apparent from these figures that dependence below 6 months of administration has, in the vast majority of instances, been reported at higher doses and usually with cross-reacting substance use. An exception is discussed later. However, with continuous use for more than 6 months there are now a substantial number of reported cases at accepted therapeutic dose levels, As Petursson and Lader (1984) have pointed out, the withdrawal reaction that occurs after prolonged use of therapeutic dosage may be as severe as that after high dosage under abuse conditions.

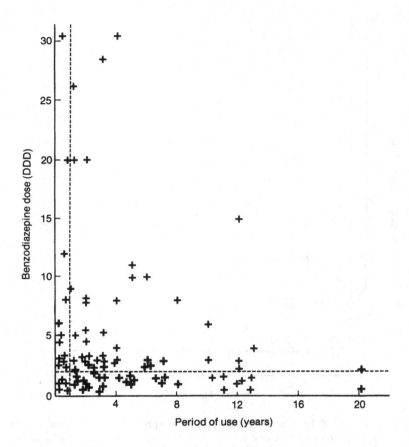

Figure 5 Analysis of the dose of benzodiazepine (expressed in DDD) and length of use for those not reported to be using alcohol and/or drugs. The lines parallel to the ordinate and abscissa represent DDD×2 and 6 months, respectively

Drugs involved

Nearly all benzodiazepines that have been available commercially for some time are implicated (Table 2). There is no indication that the clinical profile of the substance alters the dependence risk. It should be noted that this applies to both 1,4- and 1,5-benzodiazepines, and also that it is fallacious to believe that short-acting compounds have a lower risk. Indeed it is clear from several publications that the short-acting and rapidly acting compound lorazepam *may* have a higher dependence risk relative to the extent of its use. This is discussed later.

The only exceptions that may exist to the view that all benzodiazepines

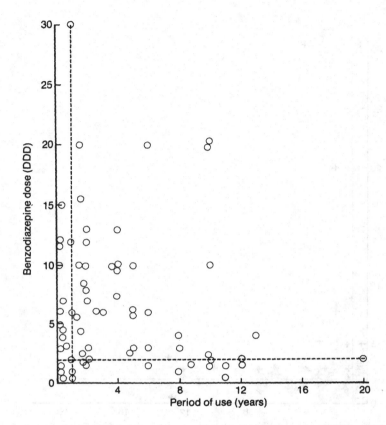

Figure 6 Analysis of the dose of benzodiazepine (expressed in DDD) and length of use for those reported to be using alcohol and/or drugs. The lines parallel to the ordinate and abscissa represent DDD×2 and 6 months, respectively

are involved are the ultra-short-acting compounds (half-life probably under about 6 hours). While there *may* be daily rebound reactions with these compounds, particularly in high dosage, and disinhibition reactions have been seen, classical physical dependence with withdrawal phenomena currently appear to be encountered less than would be expected.

Tolerance

Reference has already been made to the very rare group of cases in which there is a pure dependence on very high doses of one of the benzodiazepines. Such patients show negligible effects (e.g. sedation, ataxia) from these high doses and have clearly developed a large measure of tolerance.

Table 2 The benzodiazepines for which there is clear evidence of the development of withdrawal symptoms

Anxiolytic		Muscle relaxant		Hypnotic	
Diazepam	440	Clonazepam	6	Nitrazepam	22
Chlordiazepoxide	193			Flunitrazepam	7
Lorazepam	39			Flurazepam	2
Oxazepam	32			Temazepam	1
Clorazepate	5				
Clobazam	4				
Bromazepam	3				
Alprazolam	2				

Remaining cases either involved multiple benzodiazepines or were not capable of analysis

The common finding that the initial drowsiness rapidly wears off during benzodiazepine therapy also suggests some receptor tolerance. That this tolerance occurs at receptor sites rather than involving pharmacokinetic changes, has been demonstrated (Petursson and Lader, 1984). Petursson and Lader (1984) have also produced pharmacological evidence of tolerance even when continued anxiolytic effect is achieved with no dose elevation.

However, while there is rapid tolerance to the sedative effect there is usually no apparent clinical tolerance to the anxiolytic effect. As Hollister *et al.* (1980), among many others, have pointed out, long-term therapy is effective with no dosage increase in most cases. There is, moreover, probably no enzyme induction under clinical conditions (Greenblatt and Shader, 1974). On the other hand previous tolerance to sedatives and/or alcohol does seem to encourage tolerance to benzodiazepines (Greenblatt and Shader, 1974).

Since increasing dosage favours earlier dependence, the factors that lead to tolerance in some patients require further study. However, even with no tolerance, and hence effective long-term therapy at normal dosage, dependence occurs in a small proportion of patients.

Rate of elimination

Reference has already been made to the fact that dependence has been reported to occur with nearly all benzodiazepines that have been available for some time.

The interval between the time of sudden drug withdrawal and the onset of the abstinence reaction clearly varies with the beta half-life of the compound, though less active metabolites may cloud the issue. Hollister (1980) has suggested that the severity of the reaction may be greater with sedative compounds (predominantly the barbiturates) with a beta half-life of about 12 hours. Whether this is true for the benzodiazepines has still to be established.

A further factor is interesting clinicians, and this factor is revealed by the literature analysis. For lorazepam, not only is the abstinence syndrome more florid and seen earlier after discontinuation, but evidence of dependence appears to be encountered with shorter periods of therapeutic exposure in patients only exposed to the single benzodiazepine. Thus, many of the cases reported with lorazepam have occurred at dosage levels at or only just above the accepted therapeutic range. No less than 7 of the 21 (33%) have been recognized within the first year of therapy, and 4 have occurred after less than 3 months' treatment. By contrast only 9 (<15%) of the 63 diazepam cases analysed were with less than 1 year's continuous administration (Figure 7). The information would appear to demand further careful study by a prospective short-term comparative trial.

Spencer (1981) has postulated that short beta half-life benzodiazepines would be expected to show this effect since the rate at which the compound would be released from the receptor site might be more rapid than the rate of replacement of the unknown natural ligand. While this is a tempting theory it may not represent the whole story, as there appear to be differences in the propensity for producing dependence among drugs with comparable beta half-lives (cf. oxazepam and lorazepam). It may be that this is due to the rapidity of onset of the effect as perceived by the patient. Certainly it is a further indication that the beta half-life is not the sole determinant of clinical effects.

Incidence during therapeutic use

I previously suggested on the basis of reported cases that dependence on benzodiazepines was a rare phenomenon (Marks, 1978). Reported cases cannot be regarded as a valid representation of the true level of dependence, and I suggested that studies in which patients were deliberately withdrawn from therapeutic doses of benzodiazepines would be desirable. Several of these studies have now been undertaken (see Appendix 2). Objections to the details of the trial design (p. 128) can be made against each of these studies. Nevertheless, they indicate broadly the incidence of reactions to abrupt withdrawal and represent the only experimentally determined incidence as opposed to *ex cathedra* statements.

The withdrawal phenomenon itself is not necessarily an indicator of dependence as defined by the World Health Organization (1950) (Table 3). For example, the 'crutch' phenomenon is seen with other drugs with no dependence liability, e.g. glyceryl trinitrate in patients with angina pectoris. The rebound reaction is also seen with many other drugs with no recognized dependence liability (Lupolover et al., 1982). Media

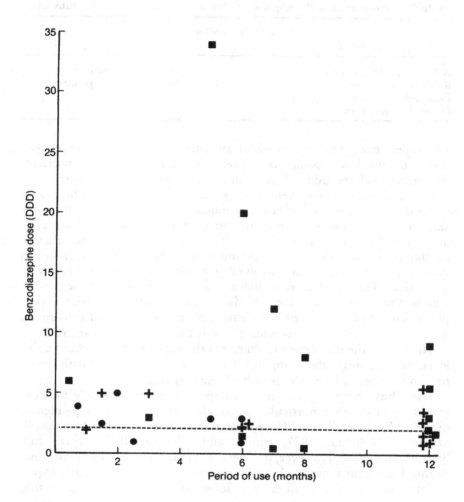

Figure 7 A more detailed analysis of the cases in Figure 5, in which abstinence occurred after only a short course of treatment ● lorazepam; ■ diazepam; + other benzodiazepines

anecdotal publicity has given rise to an expectation of withdrawal effects, and cases of 'pseudo-dependence' have been described when patients in controlled withdrawal trials were in fact continued on the benzodiazepine. The recurrence of the anxiety state is usually more easily recognized, for the return of symptoms typically occurs later than those related to dependence, and they persist and even increase in severity rather than receding.

Hence, it is important to appreciate that only a proportion of those

Table 3 Classification of the response to abrupt withdrawal of sedative substances

Withdrawal	Majority no problems	Craving
Rebound anxiety/insomnia		Crutch phenomenon
Return of anxiety state		Psychological dependence
Pseudo-dependence		
Physical dependence		

who experience symptoms on withdrawal are suffering from true psychological or physical dependence. Nevertheless for the patient concerned, the withdrawal reaction is just as unpleasant whatever the cause.

On the basis of the current studies some conclusions may be drawn about the incidence of withdrawal phenomena when long-acting benzodiazepines are administered on a continuous basis. Below 3–4 months the incidence of clinically recognizable dependence is virtually nil (though special tests *may* indicate its development at an earlier stage) unless there are additional factors involved (e.g. alcoholism, use of sedatives/ hypnotics). Thereafter there is such a large variation between the various studies that exact formulation of risk is not possible. At about 1 year the incidence of significant withdrawal phenomena is relatively small. Thereafter the incidence rises steeply and there is a significant risk.

The higher the unit dose the shorter is the exposure for reaching a risk level, but the single most important factor in the genesis of withdrawal reactions appears to be the length of administration.

There have been suggestions that dependence is more likely to occur in individuals with a particular personality, the so-called 'dependence-prone' individuals. The evidence suggests that this is true for the benzodiazepines (Hollister, 1977; Smith and Wesson, 1983; Tyrer and Seivewright, 1984). However, it is clear that many who become dependent during long-term therapy show no evidence of such psychopathology.

For some benzodiazepines, e.g. lorazepam, there is evidence that dependence can occur at an earlier stage (i.e. under 3 months); that the overall incidence may be greater, and that reactions occur shortly after withdrawal, and are more intense. It may be that a more important feature than length of action with these substances is rapid passage into the brain with a perceived 'euphoric' effect.

A group of ultra-short-acting drugs, some of which rapidly enter the brain, are currently under clinical study. According to the views of Hollister (1980) the maximum intensity of the dependence reaction exists at an elimination half-life of about 12–15 hours and ultra-short-acting drugs should show minimal intensity. There is inadequate experience yet to determine whether Hollister's findings on other groups of tranquillo-sedatives also apply to benzodiazepines.

8
Benzodiazepine 'street scene' abuse

As has already been explained, benzodiazepines, like almost any psychoactive drug, can be subject to both dependence and street or socio-recreational abuse. The question of dependence within therapy has already been considered (Chapter 7) and it is now important to analyse the question of the abuse of benzodiazepines within the street abuse scene. There are many sources of confusion that compromise such an attempt at objective analysis. Any drug abuse pattern is a complicated interaction of physical, psychological, pharmacological and socio-cultural variables. In the case of the benzodiazepines, as with several other drugs, one of the complicating factors has been the overstatement of benzodiazepine abuse in the media.

PRIMARY BENZODIAZEPINE ABUSE

On a world-wide basis it is clear that this is rare and in the WHO 6th review (1982), it is specifically accepted that 'very few use benzodiazepines as their primary drug of abuse'.

The international situation related to primary benzodiazepine abuse has also been studied by Navaratnam (1982). He stresses that abuse restricted to a benzodiazepine is rare in most countries and quotes as an example the admission figures for Thanyarak Hospital in Thailand where less than 1% of the addiction admissions were for benzodiazepines. He also quotes the Swiss study by Ladewig (see below) in support of this view.

In the USA, Ayd (1981) has reported that most long-term single benzodiazepine users do so for therapeutic purposes. Drug treatment programmes such as the Haight Ashbury Free Medical Clinic in San Francisco (Smith and Wesson, 1983) report that in the illicit drug culture the benzodiazepines are clearly secondary drugs. They are used mainly

49

as a form of self-medication for relief of side-effects in individuals ranging from methadone maintenance clients to cocaine abusers.

Within the United Kingdom too the number of cases of primary benzodiazepine abuse is very small indeed (Marks, 1978, 1983a,b) and is accepted by the regulatory authorities as no problem. One particular comment (Prescott, 1983) appears to be relevant in this respect: 'They are not 'fun' drugs. . . . In Edinburgh drug takers and pushers often break into chemists' shops. They are very discriminating and clear out all the narcotics, barbiturates, methaqualone and amphetamines but leave the benzodiazepines behind'.

Against this background of the accepted low incidence of primary benzodiazepine abuse, it is important to examine the few contrary statements. Thus the World Health Organization 5th Review of Psychotropic Substances (1981a) stated that there have been reports of primary benzodiazepine abuse in the Far East, and the Philippines and Malaysia are specifically named. The author has visited several countries in the Far East and in discussions with the police and regulatory authorities has learned that primary benzodiazepine abuse is excessively rare. When benzodiazepine abuse occurs it is almost always secondary to the abuse of other drugs. It appeared that the isolated reports referred to by the WHO really concerned therapeutic misuse rather than abuse. In that same report (WHO, 1981b), Thailand reported 150 cases of reputed primary abuse; but this must be contrasted with the estimated 400 000 cases of narcotic abuse in that country over the same period.

In a Canadian study (Sellers et al., 1981) it would appear on first reading that there are a substantial number of cases of primary benzodiazepine abuse. Close examination reveals, however, that though it is not possible to determine the numbers exactly, most represent either suicide attempts (i.e. single overdose users) or multiple drug abusers.

The studies have been extended by the Canadian group and are the subject of two recent apparently conflicting reports, both of which refer to 114 patients. In the first of these reports (Busto et al., 1983b) 49% were regarded as pure benzodiazepine abusers and 51% as multiple drug abusers. These two groups appeared to have different characeristics (see also p. 27), with the pure benzodiazepine abusers taking lower average daily doses (23 mg, cf. 86 mg), being older and having taken benzodiazepines for a longer period. In their more recent report (Sellers and Busto, 1983) they speak about only four patients who had used benzodiazepines alone. Both reports are very brief and the reason for the difference is not clear.

In Europe there are four reports that require attention (Allgulander, 1978; Kemper et al., 1980; Van Oefele et al., 1983; Binder et al., 1984). These cover a total of some 700 patients. Unfortunately the information given makes it difficult to assess the exact proportion that represent dependence in therapeutic use, the proportion of multiple drug abuse and those that are single drug primary abusers of benzodiazepines. Examination of the papers, however, shows that the vast proportion represent multiple drug abusers, confirming that in Europe, as in other areas, primary benzodiazepine abuse is rare.

On the other hand a questionnaire interview of all Swiss physicians to determine the incidence of abuse (Ladewig et al., 1981) reported a different picture. Ladewig's criterion of abuse is a strict one, though probably also embracing some cases that I have classed as misuse. Over 70% of the physicians replied. All those who reported observations of abuse were interviewed by telephone using a structured questionnaire. Having excluded unproven cases and those with inadequate evidence, Ladewig found an abuse incidence in Switzerland of 434 patients (Table 4). The 180 cases of primary benzodiazepine abuse in a population of 6.1 million, or as Ladewig calculated, two dependence cases per 100 000 prescriptions for benzodiazepines, is low. Risk of individual benzodiazepines followed availability and as Ladewig noted 'It was not possible to identify any increase in the inappropriate use of a particular compound. Among those found to be misused were both drugs with short half-life and those with long half-life, so that, from the epidemiological point of view, it is not possible to establish a connection between half-life and abuse risk.' This is the conclusion that I have reached from other evidence (p. 43).

Table 4 The results of a questionnaire among Swiss doctors on the incidence of withdrawal problems (see text for details: after Ladewig et al., 1981)

Benzodiazepines alone	180 patients	41%
Switch to benzodiazepines	14 patients	
Combined benzodiazepine/alcohol	105 patients	} 55%
Combined benzodiazepine/drugs	135 patients	

The primary benzodiazepine abuse cases are not associated with social, public health or medical sequelae and there is no evidence that benzodiazepine users act as agents for the spread of abuse of these drugs (Navaratnam, 1982; Marks, 1983a,b; Smith and Wesson, 1983).

SECONDARY BENZODIAZEPINE ABUSE

Benzodiazepine abuse is a feature of the mixed drug abuse found in many countries at the present time. The exact pattern of the drugs that are used, and particularly the primary drug of abuse, depends upon a variety of factors which include the social class of the group (university students compared with elderly alcoholics); local and national fads and fashions; and the availability of drugs in the community. In many countries and cultures the narcotics are the primary drugs of abuse, though overall it is probable that alcohol represents a much more extensive, more dangerous and more important problem. In other areas the primary drugs of abuse may be marihuana, hallucinogenic fungi, cocaine or solvents.

A sedative is usually included within the drug mixture and at the present time this is commonly a benzodiazepine. Navaratnam (1982) points out that part of this secondary abuse should be regarded as iatrogenic since it stems from the subsequent abuse of a benzodiazepine that has been prescribed during a doctor's attempt to withdraw another drug (including alcohol). Most cases, however, arise directly within socio-recreational use.

Among the secondary benzodiazepine abusers we must also include drug experimenters as opposed to the habitual drug abusers. The proportion of these is currently unknown (Navaratnam, 1982).

THE EXTENT OF ABUSE OF BENZODIAZEPINES AMONG KNOWN NARCOTIC ABUSERS

The first report that attempted to determine the extent of the problem was that of Woody *et al.* (1975), who found that up to 40% of their narcotic abusers were 'diazepam users'. Their report stresses that a proportion of these were diazepam 'misusers', i.e. were using diazepam, however misguidedly, in a therapeutic sense. Numerous later studies have attempted to determine the proportion that are benzodiazepine users within the abuse scene.

The main method is by routine urine testing despite the fact that urine test methods are far from reliable in this group because such patients produce fake urine samples (Dally, 1983). This is in contradistinction to alcoholics, whom Busto *et al.* (1983a) found reliable in their reporting of benzodiazepine use.

Primm (1981) reported a low incidence in random urine samples of a population of heroin addicts in Harlem, as did Senay *et al.* (1977) (3%) among a group on methadone maintenance withdrawal in Chicago. Among a group of alcoholics minor tranquillizers were being used by 12.7% prior to treatment (Sokolow *et al.*, 1981). A study of 6000 Los Angeles County probationers (Budd, 1981) revealed 350 benzodiazepine-positive urines (about 6%). Of these 350, 58% were associated with other drugs, mainly narcotics. It is not clear, however, how many of the 147 urines (i.e. about 2.5% of the total population) who showed only a benzodiazepine on urinalysis were receiving them therapeutically. Cushman and Benzer (1980) found 69 (9.2%) urinary metabolite cases of benzodiazepine use in 750 consecutive entrants to a drug dependence treatment programme. Hence these studies suggest a figure of 10% or less of drug abusers who also use benzodiazepines.

On the other hand, there is the WHO report (WHO, 1981) that urine testing of patients in one methadone treatment programme gave up to 65% positive results for the simultaneous ingestion of benzodiazepines. This figure, by far the highest of any reported (as much as a 10-fold factor above most surveys) is based on a study in only 29 patients in two centres and may not be typical. Yet it is this high figure which is quoted by WHO (1982).

An alternative method for determining the level of secondary abuse is to take a careful history from patients, though this also may not always be reliable. In one such study in various USA centres on a group of 427 admissions to drug abuse treatment programmes there were 692 mentions of other drug use during the past year (several used multiple drugs) and of these there were 195 benzodiazepine mentions, though this does not indicate the proportion of the admissions who had used benzodiazepines (Brown and Chaitkin, 1981). It would, however, appear that the abuse of benzodiazepines was irregular, for during the month prior to admission there were only 74 mentions of benzodiazepines.

One of the most extensive recent reviews of multiple drug abuse is that of Kornblith (1981). This covers over 30 papers between 1964 and 1978. It is noteworthy that the use of non-barbiturate sedatives (predominantly benzodiazepines) is in nearly all instances less than that of hallucinogens, barbiturates, alcohol and stimulants among primary narcotic addicts. Specifically, contrary to the WHO report (1982), sedative hypnotic abuse was low in methadone maintenance patients (Senay et al., 1977; Newman, 1977; Perkins and Bloch, 1970; Kornblith and Shollar, 1978).

It is interesting to note that the proportion of benzodiazepine users among cocaine abusers is less than that in narcotic abusers (Budd, 1981).

THE REASONS FOR USE OF BENZODIAZEPINES AMONG NARCOTIC ABUSERS

There would appear to be three reasons for the use of the benzodiazepines in the mixed drug abuse situation. One or more of these may apply at any period in the individual case.

1. As a substitute drug when the narcotic drug of primary dependence is not available. Attention to this use is specifically referred to in the WHO (1981, 1982) reports and is also stressed in the study by Navaratnam (1982). The use of benzodiazepines reduces the unpleasant withdrawal effects from narcotic substances and is an attempt to overcome the withdrawal that would be experienced. Those who have abused narcotics extensively always stress that they do not regard the benzodiazepine as a satisfactory equivalent substitute for the narcotic

but that it makes the reduced narcotic dose more tolerable.

Some measure of the substitution preference can be determined from the differential street price, particularly as benzodiazepines are so widely available in the community that they have virtually no scarcity factor in their price. In the San Francisco drug culture (Smith and Marks, 1985), for example, diazepam sells at a relatively low price (approximately 50 cents per tablet) compared with, for example, pharmaceutical methaqualone ($5.00 per tablet).

Another factor that indicates the low preference rating for the benzodiazepines is that diazepam has been imported illicitly into the USA where it is not sold in the black market as such but is made into counterfeit methaqualone tablets which sell 'at a higher price than that commanded by benzodiazepines' (WHO, 1982).

2. As a euphoriant, particularly when combined with methadone (WHO, 1981; Preston et al., 1984). Individual benzodiazepines, when taken alone, are only perceived as being mildly euphoriant by those accustomed to drug recreational use. This euphoriant feature is only seen when the dose of the benzodiazepine is escalated above the normal therapeutic level and used with a narcotic (Preston et al., 1984). There is a possibility that this euphoriant effect may be a reason for benzodiazepine abuse among narcotic abusers in Thailand (Poshychinda, 1982) but, as the author states, the current data 'by far fall short of presenting a clear pattern of the status of the situation' (Navaratnam, 1982). It has been suggested (Stilzer et al., 1981) that this potentiating effect may be the result of altered distribution or metabolism of the methadone or of modulation of the central nervous system endorphin systems, but the mechanism involved is not yet known (Preston et al., 1984).

3. To reduce the side-effects during narcotic abuse, and in particular to overcome the anxiety state provoked by a 'bad' trip with heroin or amphetamines. Whether such use, and its extent is unknown, should really be regarded as abuse rather than misuse, is a matter for dispute.

THE BENZODIAZEPINES THAT ARE ABUSED

A study in 1978 (Marks, 1978), updated in 1983 (Marks, 1983a,b) indicates that most if not all the benzodiazepines that are readily available are abused. The drugs differ from one country to another and from one time to another. This seems to depend on such factors as the availability of the substance within the community, and to a certain extent upon communication within the members of the socio-recreational drug scene rather than any clear preference. The factor which may determine some aspect of preference is the rate of absorption from the alimentary canal. Substances that are slowly absorbed are not, on the whole, perceived as exerting a distinguishable effect, while those that are rapidly absorbed and distributed to the central nervous system appear to be preferred.

Navaratnam (1982) stressed that the information was incomplete, but on the basis of data reported to the United Nations for 1981/1982 found that 22 out of 57 countries indicated the existence of some benzodiazepine abuse, but of these only 16 suggested that there was a problem causing public health concern. The abuse involved 22 different benzodiazepines (if illicit traffic is taken as an indication of abuse). 'The data tend to indicate that benzodiazepine abuse is minor compared to the general drug abuse problem or even opiate abuse . . . several countries stressed that benzodiazepine abuse was a secondary problem component to the problems associated with narcotic drugs'. He also notes the variation which exists from one country to another, quoting the cases of diazepam in Thailand, flunitrazepam in Singapore, lorazepam in Mauritius and oxazepam in Australia. Navaratnam suggested that the prevalence of abuse bears a close relationship to the market penetration in a country of the various benzodiazepines, i.e. ready availability.

BENZODIAZEPINE USE AND ABUSE IN ALCOHOLICS

Although it has been known that alcoholics are very heavy users of sedative compounds (previously barbiturates; Devenyi and Wilson, 1971) the extent of benzodiazepine use and abuse has only recently been quantified (Busto et al., 1983a).

In this Toronto study, urinalysis in 216 consecutive outpatient referrals of alcoholics revealed 33% which contained benzodiazepine metabolites. The incidence in women (48%) was significantly higher than that in men (28%). Fifty-four per cent (47 patients) of those with a positive urine screen were regarded as abusers (on the basis of their history and urinalysis) although only one patient regarded himself as an abuser rather than a user. The benzodiazepine use was a substitute for the barbiturates which were only found in three urines.

One interesting feature of their study was that this group were reliable over admitting benzodiazepine use. Alcoholics are normally unreliable witnesses (Devenyi and Wilson, 1971; Orrego et al., 1979) as are narcotic abusers (Dally, 1983).

TECHNIQUES OF BENZODIAZEPINE WITHDRAWAL IN THE ABUSE SITUATION

So far as withdrawal from the benzodiazepine in the abuse situation is concerned, the technique is essentially the same as in the dependent patient under therapeutic circumstances. There are two separate techniques that are advocated and these are described in Chapter 9 (p. 76 *et seq.*)

ABUSE DIFFERS SIGNIFICANTLY FROM THERAPEUTIC DEPENDENCE

As has been noted earlier, there have been suggestions that dependence under therapeutic use and socio-recreational abuse are merely facets of one single drug dependence phenomenon. The evidence does not support this view (p. 27).

1. Although those who develop dependence during therapeutic use have often been dependent on other sedative substances (either alcohol or hypnotics) therapeutic dependence rarely leads to socio-recreational abuse in the case of the benzodiazepines, whereas it is an all-too-common feature with the narcotics.
2. Tolerance leading to dose escalation is very rare during therapeutic dependence but is common during the abuse situation.
3. The group of people involved with socio-recreational narcotic and secondary benzodiazepine abuse differs significantly from that of the therapeutic long-term users.

SOCIO-MEDICAL APPRAISAL OF BENZODIAZEPINE ABUSE

Drug abuse is a multifactorial and complex interaction which involves the personality of the individual, the environmental situation in which the individual is placed and the pharmacological effects of the drugs themselves (Figure 8). The pharmacological effects of the drugs are but one factor and perhaps only a relatively small one. Equally those who abuse drugs for socio-recreational purposes do not readily give up the habit in its entirety but substitute alternative drugs. They can usually state a clear preference rating for their substitution.

While it is not denied that the fundamental aim of management of drug abuse should be the total withdrawal of all drugs by techniques that take full account of the multifactorial aetiology I have doubts whether this can be achieved for a substantial proportion of socio-recreational drug abusers.

In the light of this I believe that the pragmatic approach on the drug use aspect is to attempt to encourage the *lowest dosage of the least toxic drugs.* I therefore have grave doubts from both a medical and social point of view whether so much concern should be expressed about the substitution

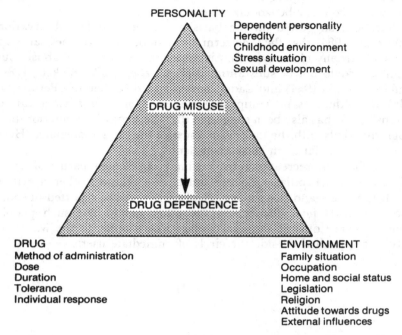

PERSONALITY

Dependent personality
Heredity
Childhood environment
Stress situation
Sexual development

DRUG MISUSE

DRUG DEPENDENCE

DRUG
Method of administration
Dose
Duration
Tolerance
Individual response

ENVIRONMENT
Family situation
Occupation
Home and social status
Legislation
Religion
Attitude towards drugs
External influences

Figure 8 A representation of the multiple causes of drug abuse (based on Kielholz, 1971)

of narcotics by benzodiazepines. Indeed I submit that any substitution of the more toxic alternative, be it narcotic or sedative, by the safer benzodiazepine should be encouraged. I fully accept that total substitution is not feasible. The policy that has been outlined elsewhere (Smith and Marks, 1985) speaks for the broader use of the methadone–benzodiazepine regime within the therapeutic community in association with all other methods that attempt to overcome the broad problem of drug abuse.

Such a policy is only appropriate if it is clear that the medical and social risks of the benzodiazepines are substantially less than those of the narcotics. It is therefore a matter of concern to find that the WHO (1981) report comments that the abuse of the benzodiazepines leads to a 'striking deterioration in personal care and in social interactions'. It is not clear whether this personal neglect refers to the very few cases of primary abuse of the benzodiazepines or to benzodiazepine abuse which comes secondary to abuse of other substances. If the latter, then the conclusion is open to considerable doubt in interpretation, for there is considerable deterioration associated with the drugs of primary dependence in the majority of such cases. Examination of the literature reveals little evidence to support the view expressed by the WHO for either primary or secondary benzodiazepine abuse.

It has been suggested on the basis of an uncontrolled observation (Lader *et al.*, 1984) that the long-term abuse of benzodiazepines can lead to cortical atrophy of the type that is associated with alcohol abuse, but this finding could not be substantiated (Poser *et al.*, 1983; Rickels, 1984; Allgulander *et al.*, 1984) and Lader himself stated (Lader and Petursson, 1983a) that 'there is no compelling evidence for or against a causal relationship'. It has also been suggested that there may be a deterioration in cognitive skills with the long-term abuse of the benzodiazepines. Here again evidence is far from clear at present.

Within the socio-recreational drug using group some measure of cross-fertilization of benzodiazepine use must be a feature, otherwise it is difficult to understand the percentage of users that are reported in some clinics. There is no evidence, on the other hand, that such people encourage abuse outside that particular circle similar to the way that narcotics are pushed outside the circle of immediate users.

Part III

Significance of Benzodiazepine Dependence Within the Community

---

9
Medical aspects

Medical care not cure

Illich (1975, 1976), with a nihilistic approach to current therapy, stressed some of its less desirable aspects, particularly iatrogenic disorders, and spoke of a situation of care not cure.

But care not cure can also be viewed in a more positive fashion. Causal therapy for cure with no undesirable side-effects is accepted as the ideal. However, illnesses are multifactorial, mental illnesses perhaps more than many others – involving, for example, environmental, personality, genetic and biochemical aspects. Hence causal therapy for cure is rarely possible.

Therapy for mental illness should therefore be based upon a plan to try to remove stress, to modify the personality, to modify symptoms or produce environmental adjustments. With these ends in mind the physician should use all appropriate methods of treatment available to him (Figure 9). Drugs are thus only one part of total therapy and should always be used appropriately.

Even with ideal therapy, however, an end-result of cure may not be possible, either because all the causative factors cannot be corrected or because the patient wants to hide behind ill health. In these circumstances care for the patient in the long term is of paramount importance.

The drug component of care involves an appreciation of the therapeutic usefulness balance.

THE THERAPEUTIC USEFULNESS BALANCE

From the medical viewpoint the value of any drug must be based on a judgement of both its therapeutic value and its safety. Therapeutic benefit exists when the level of improvement achieved exceeds the danger by a ratio which must be related to the disease being treated (Teeling-Smith, 1983). Hence the therapeutic balance involves a consideration of their clinical uses and their adverse effects.

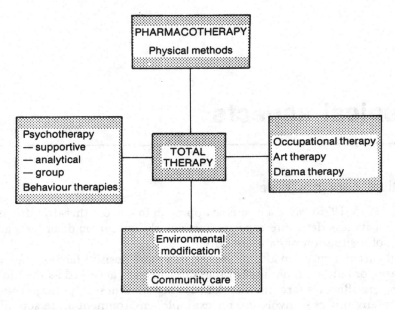

Figure 9 The concept of total therapy representing a combination of many forms of treatment

CLINICAL USES

The main use of the benzodiazepines lies in the relief of anxiety. However the pharmacological profile of the benzodiazepines includes sedation, muscle relaxation and the reduction of experimentally induced convulsions. These pharmacological properties are mirrored in the clinical activities that can be found with the benzodiazepines.

There are now over 30 benzodiazepines available for clinical use in different countries (Table 5). All the currently available benzodiazepines appear to have at least some measure of anxiolytic activity, muscle relaxation, anticonvulsant activity and sedation, though the relative quantitative activity of these components differs between different compounds (Figure 10). Dealing with each of these actions in turn:

Anxiolytic

The classification of the various forms of anxiety is a matter of dispute but one of the most widely accepted current classifications is that of DSM-III (American Psychiatric Association, 1980). The indications for benzodiazepine therapy therapy utilizing this diagnostic classification are shown in Table 6 (Rickels, 1983). They include as two of the main

Table 5 Representatives of the benzodiazepine series available in selected countries; 1984 information in alphabetical order

Generic name	USA	UK	Germany	Italy	Japan	France
Alprazolam	Yes	Yes	Yes	—	—	Yes
Bromazepam	—	Yes	Yes	Yes	Yes	Yes
Camazepam	—	—	Yes	Yes	—	—
Chlordiazepoxide	Yes	Yes	Yes	Yes	Yes	Yes
Clobazam	—	Yes	Yes	Yes	—	Yes
Clonazepam	Yes	Yes	Yes	Yes	Yes	Yes
Clorazepic acid	Yes	Yes	Yes	Yes	Yes	Yes
Clotiazepam	—	—	Yes	—	Yes	—
Cloxazolam	—	—	—	—	Yes	—
Delorazepam	—	—	—	Yes	—	—
Diazepam	Yes	Yes	Yes	Yes	Yes	Yes
Estazolam	—	—	—	Yes	Yes	Yes
Ethyl loflazepate	—	—	—	—	—	Yes
Fludiazepam	—	—	—	—	Yes	—
Flunitrazepam	—	Yes	Yes	Yes	Yes	Yes
Flurazepam	Yes	Yes	Yes	Yes	Yes	—
Flutazolam	—	—	—	—	Yes	—
Halazepam	Yes	—	—	—	—	—
Haloxazolam	—	—	—	—	Yes	—
Ketazolam	—	Yes	Yes	—	—	—
Loprazolam	—	Yes	—	—	—	—
Lorazepam	Yes	Yes	Yes	Yes	Yes	Yes
Lormetazepam	—	Yes	Yes	Yes	—	—
Medazepam	—	Yes	Yes	Yes	Yes	Yes
Midazolam	—	Yes	—	—	—	—
Nimetazepam	—	—	—	—	Yes	—
Nitrazepam	—	Yes	Yes	Yes	Yes	Yes
Nordiazepam	—	—	—	Yes	—	—
Oxazepam	Yes	Yes	Yes	Yes	Yes	Yes
Oxazolam	—	—	Yes	—	Yes	—
Pinazepam	—	—	—	Yes	—	—
Prazepam	Yes	Yes	Yes	Yes	Yes	Yes
Temazepam	Yes	Yes	Yes	Yes	—	Yes
Tetrazepam	—	—	Yes	—	—	Yes
Tofisopam	—	—	—	—	—	Yes
Triazolam	Yes	Yes	Yes	Yes	Yes	Yes

categories generalized anxiety state and panic disorder. They also include patients whose anxiety state is of situational type. Indeed it is these latter patients who form a very high proportion of those seen in the physician's consulting room.

Anxiety may also be a feature of serious physical illnesses. Patients with severe physical illness are bound to be worried: worried about the present – the ability to work and to look after the home and the family; worried about the future – whether the disease will get worse or indeed

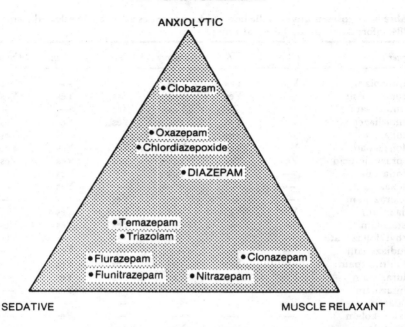

Figure 10 The activities of some of the most widely used benzodiazepines represented in terms of the therapeutic pattern

will be rapidly fatal; worried about whether there will be a permanent illness with its attendant social problems.

In its turn the emotional disturbance resulting from the physical disease can effect the physical illness, producing in its turn a vicious circle. Doctors have recognized these influences and, as various recent

Table 6 The DSM-III classification of clinical indications for benzodiazepine therapy according to Rickels (1983)

Generalized anxiety disorder
Atypical anxiety disorder
Panic disorder
Anticipatory anxiety
Post-traumatic anxiety
Adjustment disorder with anxious mood
Somatization disorders
(Other anxiety, not diagnosable by DSM-III)

studies have shown, a high proportion of benzodiazepine usage is for the relief of the emotional distress that has resulted from physical illness. Equally benzodiazepines have been used as very valuable agents in non-psychiatric patients who are under stressful situations.

Not only can physical disorders give rise to emotional stresses but emotional effects can produce many of the symptoms and signs of what appears to be a straightforward physical illnesses (Table 7). For this group of disorders the term 'psychosomatic disorders' has been used. Since the interaction is wider than this list of prime disorders we now prefer to speak of a 'psychosomatic approach' to therapy, and to recognize that mind and body are one in their effect on the well-being of the individual – the holistic approach.

Table 7   The main psychosomatic disorders

Cardiovascular
    Effort syndrome
    High blood pressure
    Angina pectoris

Respiratory
    Asthma

Gastrointestinal
    Gastric and duodenal ulcers
    Colon disorders

Metabolic
    Compulsive overeating
    Anorexia nervosa

Miscellaneous
    Headaches
    Skin disorders
    Low back pain

Psychosexual problems

The important point is that the benzodiazepines should *only* be used when distress is at a level which gives rise to undesirable body reactions. As Rickels has demonstrated (1983), the acute anxiety stress is greatly improved within the first week of therapy, and this is a very good predictor of the relief that can be expected at the end of 6 weeks therapy – the normally accepted length of treatment for acute anxiety distress.

It should, however, be stressed that while the benzodiazepine anxiolytic effect is valuable in the relief of the distress of all these types of anxiety state and of the physical ills that can result, pharmacotherapy forms only one aspect of therapy, and it is important to combine it with other methods of treatment. These include environmental modification and appropriate psychotherapy. The benzodiazepines have been shown to be particularly valuable when they are combined with appropriate psychotherapy (Uhlenhuth, 1983).

Sedative hypnotic

Of those who experience sleep problems, that is to say about one in three adults during the course of a year, about 60% have difficulty getting off to sleep, about 20% complain of waking in the early hours of the morning and then experiencing difficulty in getting to sleep again, and the remaining 20% experience both these problems.

Hence with the strongly perceived need for untroubled sleep, the level of sleep dissatisfaction that exists in the community and the initial good results that can be achieved by the use of hypnotics, it is scarcely surprising that hypnotics are prescribed widely.

A sedative benzodiazepine is now the drug of choice for insomnia *which requires treatment*. The sedative benzodiazepines may be divided into those which at the therapeutic dose produce no residual daytime effects (normally the rapidly eliminated compounds) and those that may show some residual daytime effects. The former are used where the only difficulty is in getting to sleep and when daytime vigilance is essential, the latter when there is either awakening late in the night or some measure of daytime anxiety and where some daytime residual effects are not precluded by the need for maximum vigilance immediately after awakening.

Alcoholism and drug addiction

Benzodiazepines can be a valuable help in the acute stage of withdrawal reactions in alcoholism or drug dependence. Experience has shown that by giving a benzodiazepine in adequate dosage over this withdrawal period, many of the abstinence manifestations can be at least attenuated. Such supportive therapy is particularly valuable for the patient, who is in any case fearful about the whole problem of withdrawal.

It is then important to gradually reduce the dose of the benzodiazepine in such patients after a period of about 10–15 days of treatment because too rapid withdrawal can allow the manifestations to recur. Reduction by not more than a quarter of the dose at intervals of about 5–7 days is usually appropriate.

The long-term use of a benzodiazepine in the management of the *abstinent* treated chronic alcoholic is much more controversial. Chronic alcoholics, even those who are now abstinent, have a predisposition to develop dependence on any drugs that are administered, including benzodiazepines. Chronic administration of a benzodiazepine may lead to the substitution of one dependence by another.

On the other hand there is a small group of chronic alcoholics and drug-dependent patients who cannot live in society without the support of some form of medication and in whom all other attempts at a solution have failed. For such patients, even knowing the dependence risk, the doctor may find it desirable to utilize a benzodiazepine which is medically safer than alcohol or drugs of primary abuse.

As an anaesthetic agent for special purposes

Certain benzodiazepines can be administered, preferably by the parenteral route, as anaesthetic agents for surgical procedures particularly for the relatively minor surgical procedures (e.g. dental extraction, endoscopy and cardioversion). A local anaesthetic may be added if this is necessary. As a result of the sedation and muscle relaxation the patient will lie quietly relaxed during the procedure but will respond readily to commands. Some measure of amnesia follows and this is valuable for removing the memories of distressing procedures.

Neuromuscular disorders

Benzodiazepines have been used extensively for a variety of spastic disorders of the neuromuscular system. Benzodiazepines may also be administered parenterally to relax muscles, e.g. to enable orthopaedic surgeons to correct the deformities by appropriate splinting.

The use of benzodiazepines, and specifically diazepam, has also revolutionized the prognosis of tetanus. By its use the majority of cases, even of neonatal tetanus, can be treated effectively.

Muscle spasms of rheumatic disorders and strains

Muscle spasm can be a feature in both rheumatoid arthritis and osteoarthritis. As the spasm increases so there is associated pain from the spasm and additional loss of mobility due to the contracted muscles. The benzodiazepines are of value as adjuvant therapy for brief critical periods in this muscle spasm associated with both rheumatoid arthritis and osteoarthritis.

Anticonvulsant

Diazepam is the drug of choice for status epilepticus and other severe and recurrent convulsive disorders. The benzodiazepines (often nitrazepam or clonazepam) are particularly effective in infantile spasms and myoclonic seizures. Benzodiazepines can often be added, with great benefit, to other anticonvulsants in other forms of epilepsy.

Disorders encountered in the Third World

The therapeutic indications for the benzodiazepines outlined above apply within the Third World as much as within the industrially developed countries. In addition to these, however, there are several other indications that are either specific to the Third World or substantially more common there.

Tetanus is still a very common disorder in the Third World and particularly neonatal tetanus. The treatment of tetanus remains difficult and the mortality high, but the use of a benzodiazepine (typically diazepam) has considerably reduced the mortality rate.

Cerebral malaria is still a significant danger in the tropics with up to one in every ten patients contracting malaria developing the fatal cerebral form, with children particularly susceptible. Studies from several countries have demonstrated that diazepam is very effective in controlling the seizures that are the usual cause of death in this disorder.

Chloroquine is one of the most effective and widely used antimalarial agents but unfortunately it is also a very toxic substance with a high mortality rate. The administration of a benzodiazepine significantly reduces the mortality.

Eclampsia is becoming increasingly rare in the industrially developed countries but is still a major cause of death in the Third World. Benzodiazepines have been shown to be very effective, reducing both maternal and perinatal mortality.

SAFETY OF THE BENZODIAZEPINES

Any assessment of the therapeutic usefulness of the benzodiazepines must also take into account their toxicity and morbidity relative to other sedatives (e.g. the barbiturates) as well as to the social psychotropics, alcohol and nicotine.

The estimated number of deaths per year and the crude death rate attributable to psychotropics, barbiturates, alcohol and nicotine are shown in Table 8. Psychotropics have a low mortality rate. Among psychotropics the mortality rate from benzodiazepines is even lower. 'In the medical literature there are no reported cases of fatal overdosage due to the benzodiazepines alone.' Thus wrote Greenblatt and Shader in their masterly monograph on the benzodiazepines (1974). More than 10 years later, with further experience, this is still probably very close to the truth – a remarkable record for a group of compounds with central nervous system depressant effects which have been so widely available.

One of the first large studies on the effect of overdosage with benzodiazepines was that by Lawson and Mitchell (1972). Of 941 cases of drug ingestion seen in a Scottish hospital medical unit between 1960 and 1971, 126 involved the use of benzodiazepines. None of the patients who had taken benzodiazepines died.

A further review involved a total of 773 admissions to the Massachu-

Table 8 Use and dangers of alcohol, tobacco and psychotropic drugs (based on data from various sources)

UK	Use adult (% of population)	Approx. no. using (millions)	Deaths	Crude death-rate adults /100 000
Alcohol	75+	30	8000	27
Tobacco	50+	20	50 000	250
Psychotropics	14	8	3000	40
(excluding barbiturates)	12+	7	200	3

setts General Hospital between 1962 and 1975, in which there was an acute overdosage with one or more psychoactive medicaments (Greenblatt *et al.* (1977). In 99 of these cases benzodiazepines were involved, 12 alone. Of these 12 admissions that were due to benzodiazepine overdosage alone, none required any assistance with breathing, only one was in a rather deep coma and all could be discharged without any complications within 2 days of admission; this despite the fact that many of them had swallowed between 50 and 100 tablets. In the remaining 87 cases in which a benzodiazepine was involved, multiple drugs had been taken and the frequency and severity of the complications among these patients depended primarily on the type and quantity of the other substances that had been taken with the benzodiazepine. Out of the same series, 82 took a barbiturate alone and of these deep coma occurred in 52, while 41 needed assisted ventilation.

Finkle *et al.* (1979) examined 1500 drug fatalities from a survey of 24 major cities in the United States and three provinces of Canada. The combined population totalled some 79.2 million people and covered a $3\frac{1}{2}$-year period between 1973 and 1976. In only two cases, one in the United States and one in Canada, was a benzodiazepine (diazepam) alone found to be present. In all other cases that involved benzodiazepines, multiple drugs were also involved, including alcohol and other depressants of the nervous system.

Prescott (1983) recently reported on about 20 years experience with benzodiazepine overdosage in Edinburgh. Out of some 8000 patients who were admitted following overdosage with benzodiazepines alone or with other drugs there were only seven deaths. In only one case in the 8000 'could death reasonably be directly attributed to benzodiazepine poisoning'.

Hence mortality from overdosage of benzodiazepines alone is extremely rare. In fatal cases other drugs have almost invariably been implicated. The combination of benzodiazepines with other sedative drugs, such as alcohol or barbiturates, is hazardous as there is an additive effect between the sedative components (Sellers and Busto, 1983).

The wide involvement of benzodiazepines in self-poisonings merely represents the wide availability of the group of drugs, particularly to the mentally unstable.

The safety of the benzodiazepines is all the more worthy of note by contrast to the hazardous nature of the barbiturates, their nearest rivals from the therapeutic point of view. If there were no other differences between the two classes of drugs, this would suffice to make the benzodiazepines infinitely preferable.

In contradistinction to the safety of the benzodiazepines, the social psychotropics alcohol and tobacco have a high mortality. Not only can acute alcohol poisoning be fatal but chronic alcoholism is a major cause of premature death. Although tobacco has no acute mortality its chronic effects have a risk which is even greater than alcohol (Table 9). A recent estimate suggests that at least 100 000 people die prematurely in Britain each year because they smoke (Royal College of Physicians, 1983).

Table 9 Medical and social 'costs' of the use of benzodiazepines compared with tobacco and alcohol

	Tobacco	Alcohol	Benzodiazepines
Therapeutic value	Nil	Nil	Great
Population point level of use	50%	75%	2%
Dependence risk	High	High	Low
Mental deterioration	Nil	Often high	No clinical evidence
Physical damage	Very great	Great	Nil
Family breakdown	Nil	Great	Nil
Work situation	Nil	Great reduction	Can improve
Criminality	Nil	Great	Nil
Overdose risk	Nil	Large	Negligible
Accidents	Nil	Very great	Small
Drug contagion	High	High	Negligible
Total social cost	Great from physical illness	Great from physical and mental illness	Small or negligible

So far as morbidity with chronic administration is concerned, the benzodiazepines show infinitely fewer adverse effects (Marks, 1983b) than alcohol or tobacco (Table 9).

Other problems encountered with the benzodiazepines include paradoxical reactions and performance detriments, but these are probably not common and of less concern. Reputed problems of cortical atrophy and teratogenesis have not been confirmed. The overall safety of the benzodiazepines is considerable.

While the waste of human life and happiness through dependence on alcoholism, tobacco and barbiturates is enormous, there is an additional economic loss to the community.

With alcohol, for example, this includes the support which has to be given to patient and family during unemployment and sickness, the maintenance of hospital beds and prison cells, the cost of accidents and above all the lowering of industrial efficiency. Thus, for example, the cost of alcoholism to Scotland's industry alone is estimated to be £35 million per year (Editorial, 1975) while the estimate for excessive drinking costs in the States is well over $1000 million per year (Glatt, 1974). For tobacco it has been estimated that 20 times the number of days lost per year from industrial disputes result from smoking, and that between 5000 and 8000 hospital beds are occupied each day in the United Kingdom as a result of smoking. The estimate of the annual cost to the community in the United Kingdom resulting from smoking is £280 million.

For barbiturates the United Kingdom total number of annual hospital admissions for poisoning at the height of the barbiturate availability was estimated at about 14 000 (Locket, 1973). If the cost of this care is added to the loss of industrial efficiency, then the cost to the community was well in excess of £2 million per year. The replacement of the barbiturates by the benzodiazepines has not reduced the number of suicide attempts, but it has reduced the length of time in hospital and the mortality level, producing a major cost saving.

COMPARISON OF DRUGS WITH OTHER FORMS OF THERAPY

Although the benzodiazepines' safety is good it is important to consider their use relative to other methods of managing psychiatric disorders.

The origin of almost all psychiatric illness remains obscure to us. With many conflicting theories of causation it is scarcely surprising that equally controversial views are held on the question of therapy. Most patients are likely to receive a composite form of therapy (see Figure 9) which employs the most advantageous features of a number of differing forms of therapy. These will include psychotherapy, behaviour therapy, occupational therapy, community care, autogenic training and various physical treatments in addition to drugs.

This combination of therapy, when based upon such established scientific principles as exist in this elusive sphere, is to be applauded and plays a role in the reduction of drug dependence.

Nevertheless it must not be forgotten that these other forms of therapy have their own inherent problems and that dependence can be transferred on to the therapist. Thus, for example, Hollister (1977) comments '. . .

there is no proof I know of that indicates that talk therapy, massage, biofeedback, autogenic training, muscle relaxation or any of these possible non-pharmacologic alternatives for treating anxiety is as efficacious, or safe, or as cheap as drugs'. Recent United Kingdom reviews have been critical of the value of psychotherapy (Editorial, 1984).

Little information has been published on the extent of the dependence on the therapist, and this is outside the remit of this work. Suffice it to stress that the doctor himself can influence the patients' compliance with therapy and affect, by suggestion, the influence that drugs will exert. The greater the rapport between doctor and patient, the greater is the chance of patient benefit, but equally the greater the risk that the patient will become dependent on the doctor.

MEDICAL ASPECTS OF DEPENDENCE

The level of dependence during therapeutic use

An analysis of studies that have examined the level of dependence during therapeutic use is shown in Appendix 2 and has been considered already (p. 46). From this it is concluded that if we exclude those who are drug or alcohol abusers, clinically relevant dependence is virtually nil up to 3–4 months and rare at under 6 months' continuous use. Thereafter there is such a large variation between the various studies that it does not appear possible to define the risk in absolute terms.

It is clear, however, that while there is a relatively small risk (probably still in single figures) up to 1 year of continuous use (see for example the study by Rickels, 1983), over 1 year of daily use carries a significant risk of withdrawal. However, even after many years of daily use a majority of patients experience either no problems or minimal problems on withdrawal.

Clinical implications of determined dependence risk

These estimates of the incidence of abrupt withdrawal effects are based on uninterrupted administration and abrupt discontinuation. Experience suggests, however, that few patients take benzodiazepines on a continuous basis. Either on the advice of their doctors, or on the basis of their own decisions, the majority now use benzodiazepines with an 'on-demand' technique, only taking the dose when the level of distress justifies the use (Ayd, 1981; Hollister, 1977).

Thus Bowden and Fisher (1980), for example, found that the blood levels increased and anxiety levels fell when a group who had reputedly been on regular therapy were used as the positive controls (i.e. received regular diazepam) in a withdrawal study. Others (Hollister, 1977;

Marks, 1981; Tyrer *et al.*, 1981) have experienced difficulty in finding patients with continuous level dosage for prospective withdrawal studies. Two investigations have studied the actual pattern of intake of patients compared with the pattern of prescription. Bush *et al.* (1984) found that the majority of patients (72%) use doses below those that are prescribed for them. Tessler *et al.* (1978) in the University of Massachusetts study of 236 patients prescribed diazepam, found that just under 50% followed the dosage instructions accurately, a further 45% decreased their dosage and only 6.4% increased their dosage, none to above 40 mg/day.

With this pattern of discontinuous use, the incidence of true dependence with recommended therapeutic doses of benzodiazepines can still be regarded as low, though above the previously calculated value which was based on published reports (Marks, 1978).

Reducing the dependence risk

Every effort should be made to reduce the risk of dependence to the lowest possible level, viz.:

1. By the better selection of patients for anxiolytic therapy. Anxiety is a normal emotion and serves in nature as a valuable function inducing beneficial adaptive change. The intervention of treatment merely to suppress anxiety will prevent or retard the appropriate adaptation and may do more harm than good.

   In behavioural terms, anxiety can be both a drive and a source of reinforcement. Depending on the level of anxiety relative to the task to be performed, it can improve or impair performance (Lader, 1969). For any given task the relationship between anxiety and performance (Figure 11) follows the Yerkes–Dodson law (Broadhurst, 1959). The prescription of a tranquillizer for a patient with a relatively low level of anxiety will probably impair performance and even at an optimum therapeutic level may lead to complaints of apathy. On the other hand, exhibition of an anxiolytic at appropriate dosage has its greatest benefit when the anxiety level is causing distress and is leading to a reduction in performance.

2. It is important to realize that any sedative must be used with great caution in those who have a dependence liability as exemplified by previous or current misuse of other drugs (particularly barbiturates) or alcohol. In such patients it is almost certain that dependence will occur. There must therefore be a clear understanding of the risks involved before even short-term therapy is contemplated.

3. The greatest benefit and the least harm is achieved by the careful selection of the drug to be used for the individual case. The broad question of drug group selection for diagnostic groups, or the merits

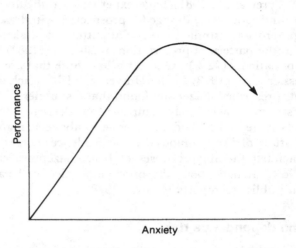

Figure 11 The relationship between anxiety and performance. The 'Yerkes–Dodson Law'

and demerits of individual drugs, is outside the present remit. However, it is important to stress that some at least of the long-term, high-dosage, therapeutically ineffective and potentially dependence-provoking prescription of anxiolytics stems from the failure to recognize the concomitant existence of depression.

4. The next concern is the method of use. If anxiolytics are ineffective after about 1–2 weeks they should be stopped forthwith.

   If treatment has relieved the anxiety it is highly desirable that it be discontinued, preferably by gradual withdrawal, after about 6 weeks and certainly before 12 weeks in all patients. It is then possible to determine whether recurrrence occurs and therefore whether long-term therapy *may* be necessary.

5. Drugs form only one part, however valuable, of the total patient care. Drugs are in the main suppressive of symptoms rather than curative. The causal therapy for the patient who is mentally disturbed by stress is the removal of the stress, not the suppression of its manifestations, and the period of relief produced by the benzodiazepine should be used to try to solve the underlying problem.

6. However, even given adequate time, it is often quite impossible for the doctor to modify the patient's reaction to his environment by changing the environment. A proportion of patients will be seen who can only exist in society with the help of anxiolytic therapy. In such patients before anxiolytic therapy is reinstituted there should be conscious appreciation that:

   (a) anxiolytic drugs reduce the distress but do not cure the cause;

74

(b) long-term treatment implies that there is likely to be a dependence problem at some stage.

There are merits in the decision to reinstitute such therapy being a joint one between the physician and the patient. The decision to use drugs again should be based on the conclusion that life in society causes considerable distress without such help. Even at this stage the lowest dose should be given, periodic trials should be made of gradual withdrawal and graded intermittent use to cover the periods when distress is acute should be the standard procedure.

7. Above all, psychoactive agents should be prescribed only after listening to the patient, assessing whether the stressful environment can be modified, what effect the disorder will have on behaviour and how best the various therapeutic procedures can be combined. However, these other procedures have their own problems (p. 71).

Caffeinism as a possible factor in continued use of benzodiazepines

Although the dependence risk is low it is clear that a certain number of patients experience considerable difficulty in stopping the drug. However the pattern of use is unusual for a 'drug of dependence' (e.g. the lack of tolerance) and an alternative hypothesis for the difficulty would have attractions.

Caffeinism, intoxication with high levels of intake of coffee or tea, is a disorder which has been recognized relatively recently. It is characterized by a constellation of manifestations that closely resemble chronic anxiety (Greden, 1974; Greden et al., 1981; Gilbert, 1976). It has been found to be associated with increased cigarette smoking (Friedman et al., 1974). Some recent studies (Downing and Rickels, 1981; Greden et al., 1981) have shown that there is an interrelationship between tranquillo-sedatives and coffee intake. The level of use of tranquillo-sedatives is abnormally high in those persons who consume more than 750 mg caffeine per day (Downing and Rickels, 1981). There is evidence too that caffeine is a competitive inhibitor of diazepam binding at the brain 'benzodiazepine' receptors (Tallman et al., 1980).

This raises the interesting hypothesis that *some* of the cases of chronic benzodiazepine use are suffering from caffeinism rather than from benzodiazepine dependence. The anxiety state which they experience on cessation of the benzodiazepine therapy is the consequence of the anxiety-mimicking effect of the high caffeine intake converted to a vicious circle by the sedative effect of the benzodiazepines. If this hypothesis is established then this particular group of patients can be relieved of the problems of long-term use of benzodiazepines by stopping the intake of caffeine.

Reducing withdrawal reactions after long-term use

Gradual withdrawal should be used for all patients who have received benzodiazepines for more than about 3 months continuously. This is particularly true when doses above the normal therapeutic level have been used. The rate of reduction that avoids withdrawal sequelae will vary from one patient to another and also varies with the dose being taken, the beta half-life and the length of administration. As a general rule *at least 4 weeks* is the minimum time for reduction and a quarter of the daily dose the maximum reduction increment. If a patient experiences problems on such a regime, then the dose should be held for a period just above the level that provokes undesired effects and the gradual reduction should then be reinstituted from this level.

It is clear that in some patients even gradual withdrawal does not avoid the abstinence syndrome. In some it is likely that a chronic anxiety state is still present and a recurrence of this is the cause. Some of the descriptions do not state the rate of withdrawal clearly and too rapid withdrawal, particularly too large increments, must be suspected. It is also clear that media reports or physician discouragement can lead to an expectation of problems. Pseudo-withdrawal reactions have occurred when patients have believed, mistakenly, that treatment was being withdrawn. The best effects are achieved when there is sympathetic help from the physician.

Withdrawal in patients with established dependence

Two methods have been described and tried extensively. With the first method a rapidly eliminated abused sedative is substituted by an equivalent and adequate dose of one of the slowly eliminated benzodiazepines. This is usually diazepam. The dose is then reduced very gradually. The rate of reduction that avoids withdrawal sequelae will vary from one patient to another and also varies with the dose and length of administration. As a general rule in cases of abuse, in which the benzodiazepine dose is usually much higher than in therapeutic dependence, at least 6–8 weeks is the minimum time for reduction and a quarter of the daily dose the maximum step for reduction. Reductions are tried at intervals of about 4–6 days and if the patient experiences a problem on such a regime, then the dose should be held for a period just above the level that provokes undesired effects, and the gradual reduction reinstituted more slowly from this level.

Harrison *et al.* (1984), in a study of 23 subjects in hospital with the abuse of high doses of benzodiazepines (18 with multiple drug abuse), used a loading dose of diazepam equivalent to approximately 40% of the reported daily consumption and reduced the dose by 10% daily. Sixteen completed withdrawal in hospital without complications and only one

76

showed a withdrawal reaction (paranoia and confusion). The remaining six left hospital before withdrawal was complete although in three of these it appears that withdrawal was subsequently completed successfully. Despite this experience of reasonably rapid withdrawal in a hospital environment, there are in my opinion advantages in the more gradual technique.

In the second method, developed by the Haight Ashbury Clinic in San Francisco (Smith and Wesson, 1983), the benzodiazepine is first substituted by phenobarbital.

Based on the patient's history, a best estimate is made of the daily benzodiazepine usage during the month prior to treatment. The benzodiazepine dose is converted to phenobarbital withdrawal equivalence according to Table 10. This phenobarbital equivalent dose is given daily, divided into three or four doses. If another sedative-hypnotic (including alcohol) is also being abused the phenobarbital conversion of this is added to the amount computed for the benzodiazepine. However, regardless of the total computed conversion, the maximum phenobarbital dose is 500 mg per day. After stabilization on the phenobarbital the daily dose is decreased by 30 mg each day.

Table 10 Phenobarbital and withdrawal conversion for benzodiazepines (from Smith and Wesson, 1983)

Generic name of benzodiazepines	Dose (mg)	Phenobarbital withdrawal conversion (mg)
Alprazolam	1	30
Chlordiazepoxide	25	30
Clonazepam	2	15
Clorazepate	15	30
Diazepam	10	30
Flurazepam	15	30
Halazepam	40	30
Lorazepam	1	15
Oxazepam	10	30
Prazepam	10	30
Temazepam	15	30

Before each dose of phenobarbital the patient is checked for the presence of sustained horizontal nystagmus, slurred speech and ataxia. If sustained nystagmus is detected, the scheduled dose of phenobarbital is withheld. If all three symptoms are present the next two doses of phenobarbital are withheld and the total daily dose for the next day is halved.

Although there is no advantage from the point of view of the psychological aspect of withdrawal, some of the physical manifestations are reduced by the administration of propanolol during the withdrawal period (Tyrer *et al.*, 1981; Lapierre, 1981; Hopkins *et al.*, 1982; Tyrer and Seivewright, 1984).

There have been relatively few quantitative studies on the results of attempts at withdrawal. One of the interesting, recent large studies in general practice is that of Hopkins *et al.* (1982), who used a gradual dose reduction technique (up to 10 weeks in practice though the original intention was to withdraw over about 4 weeks). The results depended on the length of previous use. Up to 3 years some 76%, between 3 and 5 years 65% and over 5 years 40% achieved complete withdrawal. A high proportion of the others considerably reduced their intake.

Polydrug abuse is often more difficult to manage than dependence on drugs of only one group (e.g. sedative–hypnotics). The sedative–hypnotic withdrawal sequelae may be more severe (e.g. withdrawal seizures). They may be maintained with advantage on a long-acting orally effective narcotic such as methadone while they are detoxified from the sedative–hypnotic; then graded reduction of the methadone completes their narcotic detoxification (Smith and Wesson, 1983). The presence of a benzodiazepine as the sedative component does not alter significantly the difficulty or method of dealing with the treatment of mixed drug abuse. The problem is always extremely difficult and there is currently no single or simple solution.

10
Social aspects

SOCIAL APPROACH TO MENTAL ILLNESS

In medical terms disease or illness can be regarded as a deviation from normality, the limits of normality being expressed in an appropriate statistical format.

In social terms, however, disease is not perceived or responded to in the same manner by all individuals and groups. Perception is based on value systems and sets of attitudes prevailing in the society and culture. The medical definition of illness comprises only one component of the group of values and attitudes, and the social definition of illness is a broader one. It can be defined as a person-centred undesirable deviation of one or more of a number of different measures that can characterize an individual through time.

It involves not only the physical process of the disease but the behavioural response of the individual to the disease – the sick role. This sick role becomes a mode of reacting to and coping with the existence and potential hazards of sickness. This reaction is frequently independent of and strikingly different from the criteria and norms expected by the medical profession.

Society's own criteria for health and illness vary with time and in consequence the nature of the sick role changes. Hence the social valuation of health and sickness varies with both time and social and cultural change. In line with this, society's approach to mental illness has varied.

Mental illnesses are nothing new; their descriptions can be found in the earliest manuscripts and for centuries such illnesses were considered instances of demoniac possession, with trephining to allow the demon to escape representing an accepted therapeutic procedure.

This unhappy state continued throughout the Middle Ages when mental illness was treated at best by holy men 'casting out devils', or at worst by torture and death. This was followed by the period of incarceration, at first in conditions of indescribable squalor and later in hospitals the Victorian architecture of which gave them a physical similarity to gaols. The similarity was often confirmed during residence therein.

Throughout the period there was no understanding of the nature of mental illness and even today it is only in the most sophisticated communities that mental illness is looked upon, like physical illness, as a disease and not a cause for shame. Even in current sophisticated societies the attitude is often that of suspicion, particularly among the less educated. The change towards the acceptance of psychiatric disorders as diseases resulted partly from the physical treatments of the late 1930s and 1940s but perhaps more than anything else from the development during the last quarter-century of specific chemotherapy for psychiatric abnormalities (see, for example, Pichot, 1972).

But, as Pichot and others have stressed, the very availability of psychotropic drugs has produced an ambivalent attitude within society. On the one hand there is the greater tolerance towards mental illness, but on the other a great hostility towards drug-induced behavioural changes when their manifestations are contradictory to the cultural model. Thus society tolerates certain drugs (e.g. alcohol) that are objectively extremely harmful but is less tolerant to others that may be less objectively harmful (e.g. sedatives and tranquillizers).

There are socially acceptable diseases and socially acceptable drugs with no rational basis for their selection. In our current society the neurosis and psychotropic drugs are still (25 years after their first use) largely socially unacceptable – tolerated as a necessary evil rather than lauded as a great good. Society's approach to neurotic ill-health is still broadly 'shake yourself out of it', despite the current reliance on psychotropic drugs.

Blackwell (1973) in particular has stressed what he has termed the 'puritan ethic', i.e. 'the view that patients should tolerate depression or anxiety and that medication for this end is to misuse it'. A similar view of the social approach to the use of psychotropics has been expressed by Hollister (1975) and Abrahamson (1976).

LEVELS OF USE

The first social aspect that requires consideration is the level of use. For many years now in both the British medical press (Parish, 1971; Muller, 1972) and lay press (Gillie, 1975), the view has been expressed that the use of psychotropics is too high.

There are four main ways in which the level of use of a therapeutic substance can be represented. The first of these is by the total sales level. This representation of use in monetary terms does not give a reliable indication from the medical viewpoint since it takes no account of price differences and need not be considered further.

The second method, which is the one that has been used most extensively, is based on audits of prescriptions. Since a prescription can be for a short or long period even in the same patient, let alone from one practice to another or one country to another, caution must again be exercised over the interpretation of the findings.

In an earlier publication (Marks, 1978) I estimated that in the United Kingdom there was a compound increase of growth of about 2% per year over the period 1960–1975. A major part of this growth was at the expense of the older, less effective and more dangerous compounds, particularly the barbiturates. Evidence from the United States showed that the peak of tranquillizer prescriptions was reached there in 1975 (Rickels, 1983), while in many European countries the peak appears to have been reached during the 1970s (Boethius and Westerholm, 1976). In the United Kingdom too the level has now started to decline (Marks, 1982) although the rise continued for longer than in many countries (Figure 12).

However, raw data on prescriptions take no account of the different drugs that are used in each country and the pattern of their use. The Food and Drugs Administration has, over the years, retarded the introduction of drugs into the United States of America; sometimes for good, sometimes to the detriment of patient care. Other countries have developed members of the benzodiazepine series to a different extent and at a different rate. Moreover varying patent laws and their varying interpretation by the courts have meant that the number of copies of the original drugs has varied between countries. One of the difficulties for those treating international travellers, or concerned with international therapeutics, is the availability of different therapeutic substances in different countries and the different trade names under which they may be prescribed. In a

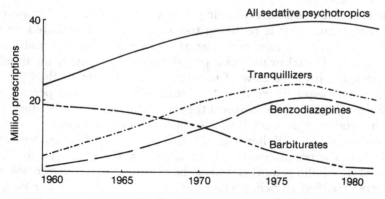

Figure 12 Level of prescription of sedative psychotropic substances in the United Kingdom (1960–1983), based on various government and other statistics

81

rapidly growing series like the benzodiazepines it is impossible to produce an accurate up-to-date list of all the available preparations. Table 5 therefore only indicates the commercial availability of representatives of the series in selected countries. It demonstrates why it is difficult to interpret figures of use and misuse from one country to another.

Because of the variation from one country to another, the World Health Organization has now adopted a new method of expressing the level of use, and this new method has much to commend it. This expresses the level of use in terms of 'defined daily doses' (DDD) per year per 1000 population (Lunde *et al.*, 1979). This is particularly valuable when comparisons are to be made from one country to another and from one year to another, particularly when the substances that are being used change significantly with time or a different prescribing pattern is adopted. However even with DDD international comparisons may not be reliable because patient audits show that the average dose used in different countries may vary markedly from the DDD.

The figures for the consumption of benzodiazepines for several west European countries for the 1960s and 1970s, expressed in terms of the DDD, are shown in Figure 13. It will be seen that Iceland and Northern Ireland have high use of the benzodiazepines with a lower use in Czechoslovakia and the main Scandinavian countries. With the possible exception of Iceland, the consumption of the benzodiazepines became level or began to fall slightly in the late 1970s. However any conclusions about the level of drug *use* that are based solely on sales volume or prescription audits may not be reliable. There is now considerable evidence from the USA and the UK that patients actually consume far less tranquillizers than are prescribed (Bowden and Fisher, 1980; Bush *et al.*, 1984; Tessler *et al.*, 1978). The proportion consumed in other countries has not been established, so that this may introduce a variable inaccuracy from one country to another.

The fourth method for expressing the level of use is by the proportion of the population that is receiving the drug. This can be based on the proportion that have used the drug at all over a defined period (often during the past year) or the point prevalence of use (namely the number that are using it at the time of the study). The former method gives a significantly higher figure than the latter. The longer the period over which the incidence is determined the higher the figure, and some errors of interpretation can occur if this is not taken into account.

In the early 1970s (Balter *et al.*, 1974; Parry *et al.*, 1973), between 10% and 17% of the population in several countries in Europe and the USA had used tranquillo-sedatives during the previous year. Between 3% and 8% were classified as being regular users, which implied a use for over 1 month. Benzodiazepines represented about 60% of this use. Tranquillizers were prescribed for about twice the proportion of women as men,

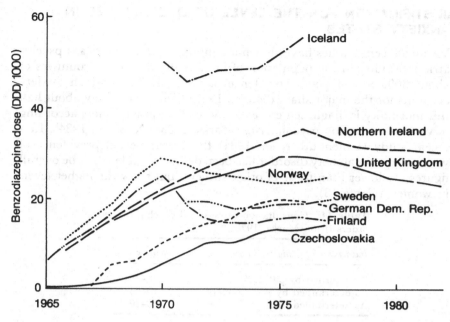

Figure 13 Level of benzodiazepine use (expressed in terms of DDD per 1000 adult population) in various European countries, based on various statistics including those of Blaha and Brickmann (1983)

and the elderly were higher users than the young (Lader, 1980b; Mellinger and Balter, 1981; Marks, 1980; Jones *et al.*, 1984).

The favoured benzodiazepines and the exact form in which they were prescribed varied from one country to another. Thus in Spain, for example, a significant proportion received fixed combinations including the benzodiazepines (LaPorte *et al.*, 1981), whereas combinations would be an exception in Anglo-Saxon and Nordic countries.

The American group who undertook the major studies in the early 1970s repeated their survey in 1979, and have reported their observations in various papers over the past few years (Mellinger and Balter, 1981; Mellinger *et al.*, 1984a,b; Balter *et al.*, 1984). They confirmed the work of others, that the level of tranquillizer use has fallen. In 1979 some 11% of the total sample had used anxiolytics one or more times during the past 12 months. Benzodiazepines accounted for 84% of this use. In part these will be prescribed for anxiety states presenting as such, in part for insomnia, but in considerable measure for physical disorders in which it is believed that anxiety is a significant aspect of the genesis of the disorder. Currently the annual level of benzodiazepine use for anxiety-associated disorders appears to be about 6%.

The level of long term use is considered separately in Chapter 12.

83

JUSTIFICATION FOR THE LEVEL OF OVERALL USE IN ANXIETY STATES

Various recent studies have shown an annual level of significant psychiatric morbidity in the population of industrially developed countries of about 30% and a point prevalence of about 15%, of which anxiety accounts for the major share (Marks, 1980) (Table 11). Only about half this morbidity is diagnosed correctly by medical practitioners according to various studies by psychiatrists (Marks, 1983a; Nabarro, 1984). In a recent study (Uhlenhuth et al., 1984) the 1-year period prevalence of various types of anxiety disorder has been defined (Table 12). The overall figures are lower than those of other surveys, but show the higher levels in women (Table 13).

Table 11 Consultation rates for all psychiatric disorders (from Marks, 1978)

Incidence of psychiatric illness	Proportion (%)
As recorded by patients	30–35
As determined by practitioners	10–23
As determined by psychiatrists	16–30

Table 12 The proportion (%) of the general public (based on 3161 sample) with various anxiety patterns during a 12-month period (based on Uhlenhuth et al., 1984)

Disorder	Total	Men	Women
Agoraphobia/panic states	1.2	0.5	1.8
Other phobias	2.3	1.3	3.1
Generalized anxiety	6.4	4.4	8.0
Total	9.9		

Hence the current level of prescription of compounds to help to relieve anxiety (annual level about 6%) is rather low to judge from this level of morbidity, even if we only consider the most recent survey (Uhlenhuth et al., 1984).

In the developing world studies have suggested a similar frequency of psychiatric morbidity (Harding et al., 1980; Harding and Chrusciel, 1975), while in Hong Kong the incidence of neuroses among Chinese new patients has now risen to some 30–40% from a previous figure of some 10%, bringing it into line with many Western nations (Lo, 1981).

The increase in the use of tranquillizers with increasing age has already been noted. This corresponds to the finding by Salkind (1981) that there is general increase in the level of anxiety with age, and that the *mean* figure for the anxiety level for those over 54 years of age is itself at a level that represents clinically significant anxiety. Table 13 shows a

Table 13 Comparison of the age distribution of users of benzodiazepines (based on Mellinger and Balter, 1981) with the incidence of anxiety distribution by age (based on Salkind, 1981)

	Age (years)		
	18-34	*35-49*	*50+*
Prevalence of past year use of anxiolytics	6.3%	12.5%	15.8%
	16-34	*35-54*	*55+*
Mean anxiety (MAI) score	11.7%	13.8%	16.8%

comparison of the recent Mellinger and Balter (1981) incidence of use by age and the Salkind mean anxiety score by age. The rise in each with age is apparent.

However, the finding that the proportion of the patients who receive a group of drugs corresponds to the proportion of the population with the disorder does not indicate that the correct patients are being treated. There is further evidence of valid use in the case of the tranquillizers. In a careful study in Pennsylvania, Hesbacher et al. (1976) examined the 'illness–treatment fit' of over 1000 patients treated in general practice. Of patients diagnosed as having no emotional disorders, 99.1% had never received tranquillizers. On the other hand of those diagnosed as suffering from or having suffered from emotional illness during the previous 2 years, over half had never had any treatment with psychoactive drugs (Figure 14). In a separate study Uhlenhuth et al. (1978) showed that the level of tranquillizer use correlated well with the level of anxiety. The US National Institute of Mental Health sponsored a study of medication use and psychic distress in a nationally representative sample of US adults. This showed that virtually all of the regular users of psychother-apeutic drugs reported some psychic distress or life crises. On the other hand, of those reporting both a high level of emotional distress and of life crises only 35% of the women and 21% of the men had used any psychoactive medication at any time in the previous year (Mellinger et al., (1978) (Figure 15).

From the 1979 US survey (Mellinger et al., 1984b) it emerged that just 40% of users showed a high psychic distress level compared with 16% of non-users. The group of users also showed a higher level of somatic illness during the previous year (19% with four or more health problems compared with 5% among the non-users), and over twice the number of physician consultations. A further indication that use correlated well with medical need was that the prevalence of anxiety syndromes was higher in women than men (Uhlenhuth et al., 1984).

Pihl et al. (1982) defined the high users as being *inter alia* older,

85

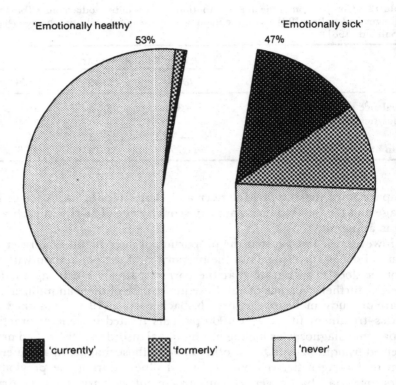

'Emotionally healthy'
53%

'Emotionally sick'
47%

■ 'currently'   ▨ 'formerly'   ▢ 'never'

Figure 14 Percentage of patients with and without emotional illness who have never received, previously received or are currently receiving psychotropic drugs (from Ward, 1980, based on data in Hesbacher *et al.*, 1976)

and that they reported being in poorer health, visited physicians more frequently (and more frequently for undefined reasons), and rated themselves as more unhappy. Pihl *et al.* suggested that both social and psychological factors are involved in the higher level of medication.

However, this still leaves the question that some of the users have a *low* level of psychic distress (Mellinger *et al.*, 1984b). It is in this group that we should consider that the risk may outweigh the benefits (Morgan, 1984). However, it is difficult to be dogmatic about this for it is difficult to be certain that these patients would not have been more anxious if anxiolytic therapy had not been prescribed.

The finding that in most developed countries women are twice as likely as men to be treated with tranquillizers (Bass, 1981; Mellinger and Balter, 1981; Jones *et al.*, 1984) has also been subjected to critical examination recently. It is clear that women report more symptoms of both physical and mental illness and utilize practitioner and hospital

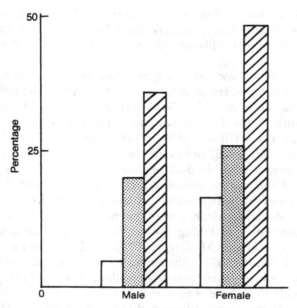

Figure 15 Correlation of the use of psychotropic agents with the level of psychic distress (based on Uhlenhuth *et al.*, 1978). Open columns = low anxiety; dotted = medium anxiety; cross-hatched = high anxiety

services at higher rates than do men (Roskies, 1978). Moreover women are more willing to talk about their emotional problems (Verbrugge, 1978; Jenkins, 1975). In the National Institute of Mental Health study (Mellinger *et al.*, 1978) about 33% of women were rated 'high' on a psychic distress index compared with only 20% of men. A similar difference was found in the later study (Uhlenhuth *et al.*, 1984).

There is, moreover, evidence that the level of prescription of tranquillizers for women who report with emotional problems is higher (Bass and Baskerville, 1981; McCranie, 1978; Manheimer *et al.*, 1973), but this is also true for those who are treated by female doctors (Hasday and Karch, 1981; McCranie, 1978). This destroys the sexist theory for the higher prescription level. Hence there is justification for the argument that the level of use in women is not too high but that the level in men is too low. With increased use, problems like alcoholism and absenteeism, in both of which there is a significant emotional factor, might be reduced.

However, before deciding that the prescribing practices of physicians are reasonable so far as benzodiazepines are concerned it is important to make sure that their use is not reducing the search for social solutions for stress disorders (Koumjian, 1981). Sociologists have also claimed that people are being prescribed drugs which they do not need (Twaddle and Sweet, 1970) and that there may be a recent shift in cultural values, whereby stoicism in the face of discomfort is no longer a fashionable virtue (Cohen, 1976). Unfortunately there have been few studies that have examined (Marks, 1983a,c) the social implications of the use of tranquillizers.

The evidence that is available suggests that there are beneficial social effects from the use of tranquillizers both at work (Proctor, 1981) and in the circumstances of general life (Whybrow et al., 1982). Moreover there is little evidence in the United Kingdom that tranquillizers are being given for social ills (Williams et al., 1982), and a study in the United States (Tessler et al., 1978) indicated that most patients are anxious to reduce their use, a sensible and realistic approach. The sociological implications of the use of tranquillizers must be viewed against the alternative means by which society deals with its stresses. There is evidence that drinking alcohol may be practised as a form of self-medication alternative to taking prescription tranquillizers, at least as far as males is concerned (Mellinger, 1978). In this respect it is salutary to note that in Finland, allegedly as the result of publicity and altered prescribing procedures, there was a fall in the use of psychotropic drugs. Coinciding with this there was a rise in the consumption of alcohol, suggesting that there was substitution of one drug by another (Idanpaan-Heikkila, 1979) (Figure 16).

Hence there is no evidence of undesirable sociological consequences from the current level of tranquillizer prescriptions, although further and more extensive studies are desirable.

The concept that their administration retards social solutions would be more valid if it could be demonstrated that withholding benzodiazepines encouraged social solutions. As Mellinger (1978) has pointed out, those in distress who are refused treatment seek solace elsewhere, and he notes that 'society often does not provide a great deal in the way of viable alternatives that are much better'.

Viewed overall, therefore, we may conclude that current tranquillizer use is medically and socially valuable: that 'benzodiazepines are far more beneficial than harmful' (Greenblatt and Shader, 1981). As Morrison (1974) put it: 'Rational responsible use of psychotropic drugs to relieve even ill-defined psychological disorders should not be considered as a craven surrender to human weakness. There is nothing really noble about needless suffering'. While this is the overall conclusion, there still remain worries about the question of long-term use. Long-term use is considered separately in Chapter 12.

This leaves open the question of the justification for the use of the benzodiazepines in the relief of insomnia. At a Consensus Development Conference in November 1983 at the National Institutes of Health, Bethesda, it was concluded that when hypnotic therapy is indicated the benzodiazepines are to be preferred to the barbiturates not only because

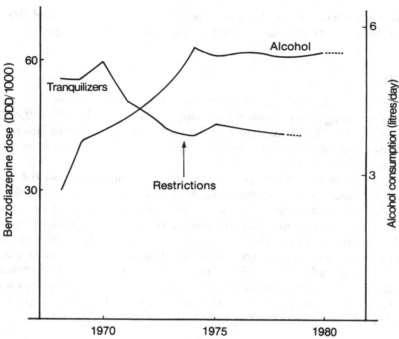

Figure 16 Comparison of psychotropic drug use and alcohol consumption in Finland

of their safety but also because of their therapeutic usefulness. The panel emphasized that patients should always receive the smallest possible dose for the shortest clinically necessary time. The general conclusion of those participating was that these substances are in general used correctly by the medical profession and sensibly by patients.

But the finding that there is negligible bad use, at least in the United States, is not enough. For benefit/risk measurement of the social aspects we must also try to find out whether there is social detriment from insomnia *as encountered in practice*, and whether this is corrected by the use of hypnotics. Experimental studies (Johnson, 1969; Morgan, 1974) demonstrate that sleep deprivation for one night produces little performance loss, but that the performance loss increases with longer sleep deprivation and is most marked when the subject is faced with boring repetitive tasks. Social studies in clinical practice, for example at work, however, are almost entirely absent and this is an area in which there is inadequate scientific information for a valid measurement and a need for further research. Among aspects that need further study are: the abuse of other substances; a failure to cope, either at work (e.g. absenteeism, performance detriment) or at home (e.g. family social breakdown); mental breakdown with anxiety, depression or psychosomatic illness.

The question of the use of any therapeutic method for the relief of *chronic* insomnia is a more difficult problem and is considered in Chapter 12.

MISUSE

In addition to this level of justified use, there is some misuse.

First the drugs may be used for inappropriate disorders. Specifically there is clear evidence that some of the poor results are due to failure to recognize and treat appropriately the depressive component of a coexisting anxiety/depression.

Second there may be inappropriate use of tranquillizers as the sole means of therapy. Any psychoactive drug forms one component only of total therapy, and their use does not preclude the need to provide all other forms of treatment which are appropriate for the particular patient.

Third there is evidence that the drugs can be used for too long a period. It is essential that these drugs should be withdrawn as soon as they are no longer required for therapeutic purposes (Marks, 1981). The amount of long-term use differs from one country to another. For example, there is evidence of inappropriate long-term prescribing in the United Kingdom (Marks, 1983a). This matter is considered further in Chapter 12.

APPRAISAL – PSYCHOTROPIC DRUGS – AN INCONTESTABLE NECESSITY

Throughout the whole period of recorded history there has probably never been any age in which people did not make use of some form of psychotropic, particularly if the broad definition of psychotropic is accepted (p. 4).

Although everyone is agreed that the best answer would be a society in which no-one needed to resort to the use of such agents, this must be regarded as a dream of Utopia, not least because some level of mental sickness is as inevitable as physical sickness and each requires appropriate therapy.

At the present time, despite a wide range of social conditions and political ideologies, there is no community in the world which has no dependence problem if we include tobacco and alcohol, which are just as surely dependence-producing. The Iron Curtain countries, until a few years ago, had remarkably little trouble from drug abuse, even though they had a major alcohol problem, but even these countries now have a drug abuse problem.

We must expect that in our non-Utopian society the majority of the community will abuse some pleasure-giving substance and that there will, in addition, always be socially inadequate personalities whose level of abuse will be well above the norm. Therefore the goals of preventive and rehabilitation programmes will have to be limited and realistic rather than aiming at impossible targets.

We must expect a continued flow of new psychotropic substances with possible ill effects for subjects with vulnerable personalities within the framework of these imperfect social conditions. While the law can be some help it cannot hope to cope with all these problems. Society in general, and its professional members in particular, should take care that inopportune concern and unduly harsh interference do not lead to an increase in the level of deviant behaviour by 'martyrdom'.

EDUCATION TOWARDS RATIONAL USE

One of the means of tackling the problems of misuse, overuse and abuse of psychoactive drugs is by education. It is essential that this should include not only the illicit 'drugs' but those generally accepted by society, e.g. alcohol and cigarettes, for there is no fundamental difference between the groups – those prescribed by the doctor, those traditionally accepted by society and those that are truly illicit. Under certain circumstances and when taken to excess, all are dangerous. What is regarded as 'deviant' behaviour today by some societies is regarded as normal behaviour by others, or normal behaviour by all in a different generation. Tobacco and alcohol are no less dangerous just because they are freely available. Hence educational programmes should deal with all types of drugs from tobacco and alcohol, through barbiturates and tranquillizers to heroin and LSD, but should give some indication of the degree of danger of each.

Education of an appropriate character must be directed separately to doctors and to the general public.

Doctors should be taught, *inter alia*, the place of the drugs within the total treatment of the patient, their merits and demerits, and perhaps above all the methods by which maximum benefit can be achieved with minimal problems. This education should also include alternative methods for the relief of these symptoms (Skinner, 1984).

Education for the general population is far more difficult, for it must aim at a change in the social pattern of behaviour, a problem that is currently occupying the minds of legislators, theologians and pedants the world over. The fact that it is a difficult problem in no way justifies abandonment of efforts to find a solution.

11
Legal aspects

The legal approach to the problem of alcoholism and drug abuse consists almost entirely in deprivation and punishment. Access to such substances is limited by controls applied to their distribution and sale.

Such measures may be taken by local and regional authorities, on a national basis or internationally, and theoretically are based on universally accepted and applied rules by all governments. However this goal of uniform and universal international control has not even been achieved for the narcotics.

In the light of this it is important to examine the criteria that exist for subjecting a substance to drug control. While these differ from country to country for national and local control procedures, there are general international criteria defined by the World Health Organization for international control.

The World Health Organization view has been expressed on several occasions, notably in 1969 (WHO, 1969)

> the decision on the need for control must be based upon evaluation of the risk; this may lead to a recommendation for control at the national or international level depending upon the interpretation of 'local area', seriousness of adverse effects, degree of communicability and the extent of illicit traffic.

> The situation will apply particularly to abuse of drugs for which there is no essential medical need.

> The kind and degree of control of a given drug are related to the degree of its acceptance, the nature of use and abuse and the degree of hazard to public health.

> Sound decisions on control measures can be taken only if reliable and comprehensive data are available. Very often the quality and quantity of information are inadequate.

In 1971 a new international convention for the control of drugs that are liable to abuse, but which did not meet the strict criteria of the existing narcotics convention, was adopted in Vienna following extensive discussion (UNO, 1971a). This 1971 Convention complements the existing legislative and control measures for narcotics, is concerned with the psychoactive substances and is known as the United Nations Convention on Psychotropic Substances, 1971. This Convention entered into force on 16 August 1976, when it had been signed by 40 governments, though many more governments have added their signatures since then. The signatory states are commited to formulating, implementing and enforcing national legislation which gives local force to the terms of the international convention.

The Convention itself (UNO, 1971a), the Commentary to the Convention (UNO, 1971b) which analyses the wording and provisions of the articles in detail, and various United Nations, World Health Organization and other reports (Lande, 1970; Kramer, 1978; Addiction Research Foundation, 1980; WHO, 1981a) provide valuable information on the way that the Convention is being interpreted in practice.

The conditions under which a psychoactive substance *may* be included in one of the schedules of the convention are clearly defined, viz.:

> the substance has the capacity to produce a state of dependence [and] central nervous system stimulation or depression, resulting in hallucinations or disturbances in motor function or thinking or behaviour or perception or mood.

or

> Similar abuse and similar ill effects as a substance in Schedule I, II, III or IV.

However, the scope of control is limited with the objective of protecting public health and an additional criterion is that

> there is sufficient evidence that the substance is being or is likely to be abused so as to constitute a public health and social problem warranting the placing of the substance under international control.

The meaning of this criterion and the extent of the public health and social problem requiring that control be exercised within the Convention was considered by the World Health Organization Expert Committee at its sixteenth meeting (WHO, 1969) and confirmed at the twenty-first meeting (WHO, 1978). It was deemed necessary for the drug dependence to cause behavioural problems that adversely affect others *and* to be 'widespread in the population or have a significant potential for becoming widespread'. When this applies, a public health problem exists and society must then take the responsibility for deciding on the need for the control of the drug.

Another important criterion relating to controls is whether 'international control', as opposed to national, 'are suitable to solve or at least alleviate the problem' (UNO, 1971b, p. 47, para. 8).

THE ROLE OF INTERNATIONAL LEGISLATION

There is no single cause for the development of abuse of any particular drug. Rather there are many factors that play a varying role which lies within the realm of the drug itself, the personality of the individual and the external environment.

Drug-specific factors – direct (e.g. dependence potential) and indirect (e.g. availability and accessibility which influence demand), may be of great importance. The desire to relieve personal problems constitutes an important element underlying the onset or continuation of drug misuse. Thus the ability of drugs to produce euphoria, inner contentment, excitement, or at the other end of the scale, oblivion in sleep, represent drug-specific causes of misuse.

Personality ·characteristics that appear to present the greatest risk of drug dependence are social inadequacy or psychopathology. Moreover patients with severe chronic and intractable psychoneurosis are likely to receive long-term sedative or tranquillizer therapy and may become dependent on the agent that is prescribed.

The external environment plays a vital role in the genesis of dependence. Social stress factors include poverty, boredom, urban conditions and trends in behaviour patterns. Cultural factors include the presence of deviant behaviour groups and teenager rebellion.

Legislation should try to take full account of the multifactorial aetiology. Nevertheless there is a need for further study and the WHO Expert Committee on Drug Dependence stated (WHO, 1981b):

> Recognizing the limits of available knowledge and understanding of the causes of the non-medical use of drugs and drug dependence, the Committee urged that further research be initiated to characterize those persons most vulnerable to various forms of drug dependence.

So far as the factors related to the *personality* of the individual are concerned, legislation can have only a limited role. Personality cannot be changed by legislation and the unprincipled, the weak-willed and the psychopath are unlikely to be influenced by norms imposed on them by others. Moreover the mere existence of publicized legal constraints may encourage experimentation in the young.

It is difficult to influence *environmental factors* by legislation. In so far as drug abuse represents a reaction to social change and technology, legislation can do little. It may be possible to influence certain aspects of the environment, e.g. urbanization, pollution, economics, the rights of minorities, etc., but these matters achieve scant attention in current international legislation.

The main force of drug laws has been directed against the *product-related* causes of drug abuse, and this is likely to remain the pattern. The main emphasis is placed on controls of availability of products of abuse and of their movement. However the importance of recognition, treatment and rehabilitation of those who are dependent is also recognized.

Drug abuse cannot be effectively prevented by legislative controls of drug *supply* alone. Thus for example, in the UK, official estimates suggest that the number of those dependent on narcotics has risen from 4000 to 40 000 over the past three years; while in the USA one-third of school children are using illicit drugs (Harrison, 1984).

A further aim must be to exert an influence on demand. Criminal legislation represents a costly, ineffective and ambivalent means of achieving this. Thus in addition to the controls of movement and supply, preventive measures are desirable and these are recommended within Article 20 of the convention (UNO, 1971a). Both technical and financial assistance are available under the auspices of the United Nations to this end.

THE RIGHTS OF SOCIETY RELATIVE TO CONTROLS

Criminal legislation is a form of social control which aims to contain within tolerable limits deviant behaviour. Normally criminal laws imply that the deviant behaviour damages others. Contravention of some aspects of the drug laws, on the other hand, e.g. parts that relate to possession and consumption, often affects no person other than the one who is directly involved.

Hence there is a conflict of interest between the desire of legislators to protect the health of the individual and the freedom for the individual that is specifically recognized in Article 29:2 of the United Nations Universal Declaration of Human Rights (UN Document A/811):

> In the exercise of his rights and freedoms, everyone shall be subject to such limitations as are determined by law solely for the purpose of securing due recognition and respect for the rights and freedoms of others and of meeting the just requirements of morality, public order and the general welfare in a democratic society.

This aspect is covered in the 1971 Convention, for drugs can only be scheduled if there is a 'public health and social problem' which warrants international control. This implies that the abuse by the individual has had repercussions that have extended beyond his own confines and affected society in general. In these circumstances the rights of the individual are subservient to the good of the community. When international controls are translated into national laws it is important to ensure that the rights of the individual are preserved.

A further aspect that affects the rights of society is that legislation should be equally fair to all. There is currently an irrationality about some of the controls, particularly when these are compared to the open availability of both alcohol and tobacco. This aspect has been discussed by Pichot (1972), Goldstein (1972) and Glatt and Marks (1982), among others. Regulatory authorities are not tackling the critical problems in social medical and economic terms but often concentrate on minutiae. The greatest international social, medical and economic benefit would come from reduction in tobacco and alcohol abuse, yet the arguments which have been advanced to suggest that neither alcohol nor tobacco come within the psychotropic criteria (UNO, 1971a) are not very convincing.

Legislative controls are only as good as their enforcement, which in turn depends on an interaction between factors of social acceptability and the ability of the police and courts to apply the legislation. Laws that are not broadly supported by the community cannot easily be enforced (e.g. attempts at liquor prohibition in the USA) and the greater the amount of legislation, the higher the cost and the less the efficiency of its application.

For these reasons it is considered that the less serious problems of abuse of sedatives should be dealt with by education rather than legislation, leaving the authorities to concentrate on the problems of hallucinogens and narcotics, the control of both of which has broad popular support. Even with this broad popular support, the control of both these groups is currently not very effective (Harrison, 1984).

PROBLEMS OF CURRENT PSYCHOTROPIC LEGISLATION

Variability of application

International conventions depend for their value on the legislative will and ability and enforcement facilities that exist within individual countries. Hence while the control concept will be uniform, application will vary in practice.

Some countries do not even exercise all the controls required under the Single (Narcotics) Convention and several countries that are already

Parties to the Psychotropic Substances Convention are not operating the defined controls under this newer treaty for cultural or economic reasons.

Restriction of therapeutic use

An essential feature of the 1971 Convention is that the therapeutic use of the substances shall be adequately preserved. This implies that the legislation that arises locally as a result of the Convention should not reduce authorized therapeutic use.

Although this is the clear intention of the Convention this does not always follow in practice. Within industrially developed nations, with adequate facilities, few difficulties exist with supplies for medical purposes, but in some developing countries the penal and medical resources are inadequate. In consequence, the placing of a substance in even the least stringent schedule often leads to its total removal from the licit therapeutic armamentarium while there is relative ease of availability within a 'black market' (Zarco and Almonte, 1977; Soueif, 1981).

Effects of the controls

Legislative controls can produce the opposite effect to those that are intended, and overcontrol can be just as undesirable as undercontrol.

Tight controls may cause misusers to transfer to alternative substances. Therefore it is important to ensure that too rigorous controls on low-risk drugs do not encourage movement to drugs of higher risk. Tight controls may also cause the user to withdraw further from society, founding or joining a subculture of like-minded individuals. In consequence the activity of legislators may perpetuate the abuse that they wish to prevent.

When the general public does not *perceive* a great risk – even if one exists – then the subculture may be large and enforcement of legislation difficult (e.g. alcohol in prohibition days, cannabis, cocaine currently in the USA). Legal measures which are out of step with accepted norms of the society can undermine respect for the law. If the law is violated widely and by consensus no victims complain, law enforcement officers may be forced to adopt practices which cause considerable resentment among the public.

Another significant problem of drug control is that it can lead to a drug-producing and dealing network which can also take part in other organized crime. Large profits within the illicit trade can in their turn lead to police corruption. Within this illicit trade the drug price rises and in its turn this leads to the user being forced into crime to cope with his dependence.

CONTROL OF THE BENZODIAZEPINES – CURRENT SITUATION

National controls

The majority of countries, both industrially developed and those of the Third World, now have local laws which cover control of benzodiazepine use in clinical medicine. The regulations usually restrict availability to prescription, either not repeatable (about one-third); limited in the number of repeats; or limited as to the period over which repeats may be dispensed by pharmacists. In about half the countries, in addition to prescription requirements, some form of local reporting system exists.

In about two-thirds of the countries the benzodiazepines are themselves specifically mentioned within the legislation (e.g. the United States); in the others the regulations are such that although the benzodiazepines are not mentioned by name, the regulations nevertheless apply (e.g. the United Kingdom).

In the majority of countries where benzodiazepines are controlled, the legislation applies to every member of the therapeutic group, and it is rare to find controls restricted to individual substances.

While there is considerable uniformity in national legislation in most countries, a considerable gap exists in many countries between the legal requirement and the implementation. Thus in about one-third of countries national legislation does not appear to be implemented effectively. Usually this stems from a lack of economic resources and personnel rather than from any active desire to avoid the implementation of the existing laws.

International controls

The benzodiazepines that were then available were first considered for inclusion in Schedule IV during the plenipotentiary conference at which the Psychotropics Convention was established (UNO, 1971a). After considerable discussion they were excluded from the list that would be controlled.

The 5th (1981) and 6th (1982) World Health Organization Expert Committee review of Psychoactive Substances, advised that named benzodiazepines (essentially all those that they looked at) should be placed in Schedule IV but the UN Commission on Narcotic Drugs rejected the reports – partly for procedural reasons. Subsequently, the 8th Review by the WHO Expert Committee (WHO, 1983) recommendation that 33 benzodiazepines should be subjected to international control in Schedule IV of the Convention on Psychotropic Substances, was accepted by the United Nations Commission on Narcotic Drugs at its 8th Special Session in February 1984.

Schedule IV requires that the distribution of the benzodiazepines shall be made under licence only. They can be dispensed only on the basis of medical prescription. Schedule IV also implies some reporting requirements on the quantities exported and imported.

This decision did not even cover all the benzodiazepines that were available at the time of the decision because not all were included in the review. As Smith and Marks have pointed out elsewhere (1985), this will encourage the substitution of these other substances in the mistaken belief that they have a lower dependence risk.

The author still considers that international control of the benzodiazepines is neither necessary nor desirable for the following reasons:

1. The dependence risk is low.
2. The benzodiazepines are not drugs of primary abuse.
3. A high benefit to cost ratio for control has not been demonstrated.
4. There is no evidence that international control will improve the situation beyond that achieved by local legislation.
5. There will be a reduction in availability for therapeutic purposes in some countries but illicit supplies will not be affected.
6. Dependence is most likely to occur with inappropriate long-term therapeutic administration. This can be dealt with best by educating medical, paramedical and lay people on the appropriate use of these substances.
7. Resources will be diverted from the control of more dangerous substances, particularly narcotics.

12
Consideration of long-term use

Since the therapeutic use of the benzodiazepines covers a wide range of clinical disorders (p. 62 *et seq.*) it follows that there should be separate consideration of the wisdom of long-term use for at least the four principal therapeutic actions:

anti-anxiety
sedation
muscle relaxation
anticonvulsant

ANTI-ANXIETY

Except for the most ardent protagonist of psychotherapy, there can be few who deny that short-term pharmacological anxiolytic therapy is beneficial in the acute anxiety crisis and that it has minimal risks (p. 68). Acute phobic and panic attacks are psychological disorders which demand urgent therapy. For some quarter of a century it has been accepted that a benzodiazepine rapidly relieves such acute anxiety, with negligible risk of mortality from overdosage, tissue or organ morbidity or other iatrogenic disorder. Relief occurs within a matter of hours of the first dose and is maintained for as long as the benzodiazepine dose is administered (Rickels, 1983).

There is no absolute definition of what is regarded as short-term therapy but many would accept that a period of 6 weeks anxiolytic treatment is a reasonable representation of the normal time for the relief of the acute attack (Rickels, 1983).

The question of chronic anxiolytic therapy is much more controversial: consideration of possible benefit involves the balance between therapeutic activity and adverse reactions.

On the benefit side there is a need to consider two aspects. The first is the need for long-term administration of anxiolytics for the relief of anxiety. This was specifically considered at a special meeting held in

100

Washington DC in 1980 (Marks, 1981). Several eminent psychiatrists agreed that some 30% of patients with anxiety suffered from a chronic disorder with sufficient distress to require therapy. This included certain specific groups including agarophobics and obsessional neurotics as well as those with chronic situational anxiety neurosis. This matter has been considered further since then by, among others, Karl Rickels (Rickels *et al*., 1980, 1982, 1983) who found that after initial treatment which lasted from 6 to 22 weeks, some 50% were in need of more prolonged drug therapy. In the 1980 discussion (Marks, 1981), Rickels even suggested that among the anxious patients encountered in their Family Practice Research Group, as many as 80% were chronically anxious. Rickels has recently reconfirmed these views (Rickels, 1984).

The need for anxiolytic therapy for chronic anxiety can also be examined from the viewpoint of those who are using such therapy. Thus Mellinger *et al*. (1984a,b) have reported recently on selected measurements of psychic distress among those who have been users of anxiolytics for more than 12 months continuously, compared with those who have been non-users over the past 12 months (Table 14). They showed that over 50% of the chronic users showed high levels of psychic distress (48% anxiety). This compared with only 20% high psychic distress (16% anxiety) among the non-users. Hence at least 50% of patients are receiving therapy for justified cause.

Table 14 The extent of stress correlated with use of the benzodiazepines

Extent of anxiolytic use	High psychic stress	4+ visits to doctor
Non-users	20%	5%
Under 12 months	45%	17%
Over 12 months	51%	35%

The proportion with medium levels of psychic distress was equal in all three groups at just under 30%. The question arises whether long-term use is justified in this group with medium levels of distress (i.e. about 0.2% of the adult population). Further study on the outcome of those with moderate psychic distress who are not being treated appears desirable.

Balter *et al*. (1984) also showed that 15% of those who had been prescribed anxiolytics during that past year had used them for 12 months of more, i.e. about 1.6% of all adults between the ages of 18 and 79 years. Women were still higher users than men, although the proportion of the long-term users (over 12 months – 1.6%) was substantially less than that for those who had used anxiolytics for less than 12 months (2.4%). Long-term users were more likely to be elderly than were short-term users.

This figure for the ratio of long-term users in the United States accords very reasonably with the observation in the United Kingdom of a 10% annual use of anxiolytics with about 20% still using after 6 months (Williams *et al.*, 1982). If the rate of decline of longer-term use in the United Kingdom followed that reported by Mellinger *et al.* (1984) then for the United Kingdom too, some 1.5% of the adult population are long-term users. Williams *et al.* (1982) also confirmed that the elderly are predominant among the long-term users and that the ratio of women to men is less than might be expected on the basis of all users. The study by Hopkins *et al.* (1982) would appear to suggest a higher proportion of long-term use in the UK but the selection process excludes those who were given benzodiazepines for less than 3 months. On the other hand it does show that among the long-term users (over 3 months) there is considerable persistence of use (90% beyond 1 year; 62% beyond 3 years and 35% over 5 years).

In the United States, on the other hand, the percentage of continuous long-term use is much less (Hasday and Karch, 1981; Mellinger and Balter, 1981). However, surveys suggest that the incidence of misuse is small and that the vast majority of current use of the benzodiazepines is justified both medically and socially.

Hence, on the basis of these recent studies it appears that some 3–5% of the adult population suffers from chronic or recurrent anxiety states, and in over 2% of the adult population the level of distress was high. Rather fewer than the 2% are receiving long-term anxiolytic treatment.

A further relevant aspect is whether anxiolytic therapy has a persistent effect during long-term use. There is no clinical evidence that the effect is reduced (Hollister *et al.*, 1980; Rickels, 1983, 1984; Parry *et al.*, 1973; Greenblatt *et al.*, 1981). Thus we may conclude that benzodiazepines remain effective in the long term.

The third question is whether there is any alternative equally, or more, effective method of treatment.

The first alternative for consideration is self-medication. In males alcohol is the most commonly used form of self-medication alternative to the tranquillizers (Balter *et al.*, 1983; Manheimer *et al.*, 1973; Parry *et al.*, 1973). The second alternative for the relief of anxiety is psychotherapy, but considerable doubt has been cast recently on its effectiveness (see p. 72).

The social answer to most situational anxiety is the modification of the unacceptable environment that is the prime cause. Even ignoring the fact that the cost of environmental modification may be large, no political structure anywhere in the world has yet been able to achieve an acceptable environment for all. World Health Organization surveys have indicated that the level of anxiety is high whether the country be rich or poor, North or South, industrially developed or rural. Thus, while we should agree with sociologists, from the practical point of view mankind will perforce search for a chemical relief for his worries until there is a new approach to the social problems of humanity.

So far as the risks of long-term benzodiazepine use are concerned these are those of short-term use, which have already been considered (p. 68), and those that only *arise* after long-term use.

The Lader group (Lader *et al.*, 1984) had suggested that long-term use might lead to cerebral functional loss or even atrophy, but this has been disproved by other studies (Poser *et al.*, 1983; Rickels, 1984). It is also noteworthy that in the recent monograph by Petursson and Lader (1984) this problem is no longer mentioned, which suggests that the Lader group do not believe that there is a problem with practical relevance.

There is also no evidence that the long-term administration of benzodiazepines retards the search for social solutions. Indeed the concept that the administration of benzodiazepines retards social solutions might be more acceptable if social solutions were available. As Mellinger (1978) has pointed out, those in distress who are refused treatment seek solace elsewhere and 'society often does not provide a great deal in the way of viable alternatives that are much better'.

This leaves as the sole but important adverse consideration for long-term benzodiazepine therapy the risk of dependence, which has been considered elsewhere (p. 72 and Appendix 2). There is evidence that the level of risk is influenced by the daily dosage, but more particularly by the length of continuous administration. There is a substantial risk over 1 year of *continuous administration*.

It is important to see whether this level of long-term use appears to be justified. Mellinger *et al.* (1984b) showed that just over 50% of the long-term users in their survey experienced a high level of psychic distress while 75% experienced two or more health problems during the year. Twenty-eight per cent showed a medium level of psychic distress. This suggests that somewhere between 50% and 75% of the use appears to be justified.

One worrying feature about the present use of anxiolytics, long-term, is the fact that a large proportion of such patients only receive very infrequent medical surveillance. Mellinger *et al.* (1984b) note that 70% of long-term users had seen their doctors within 4 months but this still leaves 30% who had not seen their doctors for longer than this. In the United Kingdom the proportion with long intervals between consultations appears to be even larger (Marks, 1983a) (Table 15). Even with long-term therapy frequent consultations are desirable to ensure that anxiolytic use is reduced or stopped when the stress level is low.

On the basis of these various studies two conclusions can be drawn:

1. In any individual patient there should be joint consideration between

Table 15 The percentage of patients receiving repeat prescription for psychotropics who are seen by their doctor (UK data)

	Seen by doctor	Unseen by doctor
Range	36–61%	64–39%
Mean	50%	50%

Based on Parker and Schreiber (1980); Birmingham (1978); Dennis (1979) and Freed (1976)

the physician and the patient on whether the level of distress produced by chronic anxiety is such that long-term continuous use of benzodiazepines is justified despite the high risk of dependence. This is a decision that should only be reached by and for the *individual patient*.

In this respect, however, it is valid to consider the practical implications for the patients of becoming dependent. Although there are philosophical and emotional arguments against such dependence it appears that the medical implications are small provided that the existence of the state is known. The dependent patient only experiences problems when the substance is withdrawn. There are relatively few medical indications which require urgent withdrawal of the benzodiazepine, and the discomfort of withdrawal can be at least substantially reduced if the substance is withdrawn slowly with appropriate support.

2. The use of low-dosage intermittent therapy reduces the risk of dependence. The essential nature of most cases of situational nature is that of intermittent distress with periods during which the stress is negligible or absent.

Hence the logical treatment for the majority of patients who experience 'chronic' anxiety that cannot be relieved by other means is intermittent benzodiazepine therapy. The patient should be educated on the principle and technique of intermittent therapy, and should tailor the dose within a defined maximum level, reducing the dose gradually as distress is relieved and ceasing medication during those periods when distress is not present. This sytem is currently being used successfully by a substantial number of patients.

Despite this successful technique it is abundantly clear that every effort should be exerted towards avoiding the possibility of dependence by the deliberate use of short-term benzodiazepine therapy for acute anxiety state that requires drug relief. Patients should not be allowed to 'drift' into chronic benzodiazepine use due to inadequate medical care.

104

SEDATION

While there would be broad medical support for the careful use of benzodiazepines in selected cases of chronic *anxiety*, their use in patients with chronic *insomnia* is far more controversial.

Recent opinion (Consensus Conference, 1983) suggests that in over 50% of such patients a correctable cause for the insomnia can be found by appropriate diagnostic procedures. A further proportion will respond to a course of a sedative antidepressant.

If there are no correctable causes then a combination of sleep hygiene and intermittent benzodiazepine therapy should be tried. This involves an agreement by the patient to restrict benzodiazepine use, e.g. to low dosage and only on defined occasions (one night in three or each weekend). It should be associated with substantial explanation by the physician on the nature and problems of insomnia and the principles of sleep hygiene (Nicholson and Marks, 1983).

MUSCLE RELAXATION

The drift into the chronic administration of a benzodiazepine for minor degrees of muscle spasm associated with, for example, muscle strains, rheumatic disorders, etc., is *never* justified.

On the other hand there is a very small group of patients with severe and debilitating muscle contraction, e.g spastic disorders, in whom reasonable posture and/or some degree of movement can only be achieved during the administration of an effective muscle relaxant.

In such circumstances chronic continuous use appears fully justified despite the high risk of dependence that this implies. It follows that, in such patients, if the benzodiazepine has to be withdrawn at any stage it should be done very gradually.

ANTICONVULSANT

The considerations that apply to the muscle relaxant effect of benzodiazepines apply with equal or even greater force to their use as anticonvulsants – if they are effective and relieve distressing convulsions not treatable by other substances their use is fully justified. There is an even more stringent proviso that withdrawal should be very gradual, in view of the greater possibility of withdrawal convulsions.

105

13
Practical aspects of benzodiazepine use

From all that has been written it is clear that benzodiazepines still have an important place in therapy, and that overall, the benefits outweigh the problems. This is particularly valid if the benzodiazepines are used wisely. Indeed most of the problems stem from their inappropriate use.

It is therefore important to define, in practical terms, how benzodiazepines should be used most effectively.

SHORT-TERM USE FOR ACUTE ANXIETY

The administration of a benzodiazepine is beneficial in the relief of the distress of an acute anxiety crisis and has minimal risks. Relief occurs within a matter of hours of the first dose and is maintained for as long as the benzodiazepine dose is administered.

The management of an acute anxiety crisis, however, does not consist solely of pharmacotherapy. Most acute anxiety is situationally generated and the relief of the distress should be used jointly by physician and patient to determine and remove the cause or to come to terms with the problem.

Select the patients carefully. Any sedative must be used with great caution in those who have a dependence liability, as exemplified by previous or current misuse of other drugs (particularly barbiturates) or alcohol.

As with any form of therapy, the decision to start treatment also involves a decision to stop. There are two important decision points.

1. At 2 weeks – any patient who has not improved should have treatment discontinued. A proportion of such patients will require treatment for a previously unrecognized depression.
2. At about 6 weeks – all patients should have treatment stopped. The

106

patient should be seen again 2–3 weeks after the benzodiazepine is stopped. If the anxiety has not been fully relieved the symptoms will have returned and be increasing in severity. On the other hand freedom from symptoms at that stage implies that further therapy is *not needed* unless and until there is a further acute attack.

CONSIDERATIONS FOR THE USE OF BENZODIAZEPINES FOR CHRONIC OR RECURRENT ANXIETY

Prolonged *continuous* use carries a substantial risk of dependence, particularly in those with a 'dependence-proneness' as shown by previous or current overuse of alcohol or sedatives.

In view of the risk of dependence and the fact that any pharmacotherapy in anxiety produces only symptomatic relief, long-term administration must not be reinstituted lightly. All other methods of therapy should be tried before benzodiazepines are given again. The decision to reinstitute such therapy should, whenever possible, be a joint one between the physician and the patient based on the conclusion that life in society causes considerable distress without such help.

The lowest dose should be given, and periodic trials should be made of gradual withdrawal. It is rare for chronic anxiety to be continuously distressing and graded intermittent use to cover the periods when distress is acute should be the standard procedure. Most patients find that the existence of a supply of benzodiazepine, in case there is distress, and a sympathetic explanation of the situations that are likely to provoke a return of the acute anxiety, is adequate to produce relief, the medication remaining unused but available.

By the use of these methods dependence cannot be totally avoided, but it can be considerably reduced.

WITHDRAWING BENZODIAZEPINES

There are two separate techniques that are advocated. In either technique, however, *it is very important that the doctor provides sympathetic support* for the patient over the period. The difficulties should be faced and explained to the patient together with encouragement that the problem will shortly clear. The best results are achieved where there is good empathy between doctor and patient.

In the first method a rapidly eliminated benzodiazepine is substituted with an equivalent and adequate dose of one of the slowly eliminated benzodiazepines, usually diazepam. The dose is then reduced very gradually. Details are given on p. 76.

The second method involves phenobarbital substitution. The pheno-barbital is then gradually withdrawn. This is described in detail on p. 77.

With either method, some of the *physical* manifestations may be reduced by the administration of propanolol during the withdrawal period.

Phenothiazines and tricyclic and tetracyclic antidepressants should not be given during the withdrawal period since these substances reduce the threshold for convulsions and increase the risk that these will occur.

FOLLOW-UP

Whichever technique is used for the actual withdrawal, a successful result will only be achieved if the practitioner undertakes an adequate and supportive follow-up and advises about how to overcome external stressful situations. Techniques that may help are relaxation, biofeedback or meditation. These guidelines are summarized in Table 16 (based on Marks, 1984).

Table 16   Guidelines for the use of benzodiazepines (based on Marks, 1984)

Short-term use
(a) Starting
If benzodiazepine treatment is desirable explain fully to the patient the objectives and duration of the course.
Does the patient understand that drug therapy:
     May carry a risk of dependence?
     Will only affect symptoms?
     Will be changed if no improvement is seen in 2 weeks?
     After 6 weeks dosages may be stopped or reduced?
     Within four months at most the aim will be to stop?

(b) Select carefully
Does the patient have a history of dependence on, or misuse of:
     Barbiturates?
     Other drugs?
     Alcohol?
If Yes; even short-term benzodiazepine treatment carries a risk of dependence.

(c) Stopping
In 1–2 weeks review treatment:
     Has it been effective?
If No, stop treatment. Consider clinical depression as a possible cause of symptoms.
     After 6 weeks stop treatment, and review a fortnight later to see if permanent relief has been achieved.
     If not, review other methods of dealing with the anxiety. If other means cannot be used consider the need for long-term intermittent therapy, with all its problems.

Intermittent long-term use
Is the patient suffering from a disabling anxiety?
     Is the patient only able to cope in society with the help of anxiolytic drugs?

If so discuss fully the implications of continued drug therapy.
  Does the patient understand the increased risk of dependence?
  Does the patient understand:
    Medication should only be taken during periods of distress?
  Are you prescribing the lowest effective dose?
  At periodic intervals (every 3 to 4 months):
    Review treatment
    Attempt to reduce dose with aim of achieving withdrawal.

Withdrawal from long-term treatment

Does the patient understand that:
        The dose will be reduced gradually, over a minimum 6 to 8 weeks?
        There may be symptoms similar to those which occurred earlier, but these will wear off?
        Other symptoms may arise, such as distorted perceptions. These too will wear off?
        If at any stage symptoms are worrying, a consultation can be arranged?
        That treatment will stop by an agreed date?
Dosage reduction – if problems are experienced, consider:
    Is the drug rapidly eliminated?
If Yes, change to an equivalent dose of a slowly eliminated benzodiazepine.
  Aim to reduce the daily dose by no more than 25% at each stage.
Reduce dosage every 4–6 days.
    Does patient experience problems?
If Yes, hold dose just above level which provokes undesired effect, then reduce more gradually.

During withdrawal

Provide sympathetic support.
Do *not* give either neuroleptics (phenothiazines/butyrophenones) or antidepressants (tricyclic/tetracyclic) which encourage withdrawal convulsions.

Part IV
Conclusions

14
Summary and conclusions

GENERAL

1. The abuse of dependence-producing substances involves a complex interplay between sociocultural factors, economic influences, the personality of the individual, initial disease state and the pharmacological effects of the agent. The relative importance of each of these factors varies from one age to another and from one agent to another.
2. There are fashions in abuse, and like all fashions a sudden change can occur for no clearly discernible reason.
3. The history of society in general shows a relatively constant total abuse level. The possibility of altering the complex multifactorial factors in such a way that abuse ceases altogether exists only among optimistic fools or foolish optimists.
4. In consequence the role of pharmacologists, physicians and social scientists should be seen as attempting to define agents which will be the least damaging to the individual and to society.
5. Abolition of abuse by legislation is rarely, if ever, totally successful. It can be reasonably successful for individual substances if there is public support for the measure, which in its turn implies an acceptance by the public that significant damage exists. The control which legislation implies can only be exerted by authorities on a reasonably narrow range of agents at any one time. To extend the list too wide is to court disaster.
6. Change by education must be accepted to be a very difficult task and the results generally unrewarding. In spite of this it should be attempted as the best long-term solution.

THE BENZODIAZEPINES

1. The benzodiazepines can – like most if not all hypnotics, sedatives and anxiolytics – produce psychological and physical dependence if

113

given in excessive doses over a prolonged period, particularly to patients with unstable personalities.

2. The dependence is of the type described variously as 'barbiturate' or 'alcohol-barbiturate'.

3. Dependence can also occur during therapeutic use with a time/dose relationship; the longer the time of administration the lower the dose to produce dependence. Dependence is rare with short courses of treatment. The risk of dependence may rise to a substantial figure after more than 1 year of *continuous* administration.

4. The exact level of risk during therapeutic use is difficult to establish, but is small if good medical practice is adopted.

5. On the other hand, in the interests of good medical care and economy and to minimize the risks of dependence, there is a need for greater education of doctors, viz.:

   (a)   careful selection of appropriate cases for benzodiazepine administration;

   (b)   concomitant use of other appropriate non-pharmacological therapeutic procedures;

   (c)   discontinuation of drug therapy as soon as it is therapeutically feasible;

   (d)   care over prescribing for patient who are known to abuse alcohol or other sedatives;

   (e)   all patients on benzodiazepines for over about a month should be withdrawn gradually rather than suddenly.

6. Abuse of benzodiazepines is a small problem in a few countries. It is nearly always secondary to abuse of other drugs and the level and pattern of abuse is variable from one country to another.

7. There are significant differences between dependence in therapeutic use and abuse for socio-recreational purposes. Therapeutic dependence only *very* rarely leads on to abuse with dose escalation.

8. Methods for withdrawing benzodiazepines for those who are dependent, either in the therapeutic or multi-drug abuse situation, are detailed: two methods are considered; slow withdrawal of a long-acting benzodiazepine (usually diazepam) or phenobarbital substitution and steady withdrawal.

9. When convulsions have occurred during benzodiazepine withdrawal the patient has nearly always been receiving either a phenothiazine or a tricyclic antidepressant, which are known to reduce the epileptic threshold. *Withdrawal should not take place during the administration of these substances.*

10. It is concluded that the extent of benzodiazepine dependence and abuse has been overstated by the media. Nevertheless physicians should take the possibility seriously and use all possible techniques to avoid encouraging dependence.

114

Appendix 1
Case reports

Authors	Year of publication	Age	Sex	Substance	Benzodiazepine daily dose	Duration	Comments
Lai	1961	18	F	Chlordiazepoxide	—	—	Other drugs too
Teigen	1961	—	—	Chlordiazepoxide	—	—	No additional information
Guile	1963	44	F	Chlordiazepoxide	140mg	6 weeks	—
Urban	1964	—	—	2 Chlordiazepoxide	—	—	Other drugs too; limited data
Hallberg et al.	1964	29	M	Diazepam	—	—	Poor evidence
Aivazian	1964	—	—	Diazepam	100–150mg	Several months	—
Lingjaerde	1964	38	M	Diazepam	30mg	5 months	+Alcohol
Takahashi et al.	1965	34	M	Chlordiazepoxide	60–70mg	6 months	—
		35	F	Chlordiazepoxide	100–200mg	?	—
		37	F	Chlordiazepoxide	150mg	1 month	+Drugs
Durrant	1965	30	M	Chlordiazepoxide	30mg	—	Other drugs too
Hoff and Hofmann	1965	—	—	Diazepam	60 mg	—	Alcohol too
Barten	1965	52	F	Diazepam	60 mg	3 years	Other drugs too
Czerwenka-Wenkstetteh et al.	1965	—	—	2 Chlordiazepoxide	250–300mg	—	Alcohol and other drugs
				2 Diazepam	120–140mg	—	
Lingjaerde	1965	41	M	Diazepam	150mg	6 months	Other drugs and alcohol
Anonymous	1965	38	F	Chlordiazepoxide	—	—	Other drugs too
Gunne	1965	—	—	4 Chlordiazepoxide	—	—	Alcohol involved; limited data
				2 Diazepam	—	—	
Bowes	1965	—	—	5 Diazepam	—	—	Limited data
Gabriel	1966	24	F	Diazepam	75–100mg	—	Other drugs too
Bakewell and Wikler	1966	60	F	Chlordiazepoxide	100mg	—	Other drugs too
		61	M	Diazepam	—	—	Other drugs too
Krzyzowski and Michniewicz	1966	54	M	Chlordiazepoxide	200mg	6 months	Other drugs and alcohol
Kato et al.	1966	—	—	21 Chlordiazepoxide	800mg+ (5 cases) 700mg– (3 cases)	1–36 months 8–36 months	Other drugs in five cases / Alcohol in nine cases
Marjot	1966	—	3F	3 Chlordiazepoxide	—	—	—
Slater	1966	37	F	Chlordiazepoxide	100mg	4 years	Other drugs too
Relkin	1966	20	M	Diazepam	60mg	11 days	—
Kryspin-Exner	1966	42	M	Chlordiazepoxide	c. 60mg	2–3 years	Alcohol

Author	Year	Age	Sex	Drug	Dose	Duration	Notes
Selig	1966	29	F	Oxazepam	600mg	4 weeks	Previously on chlordiazepoxide; limited data
Iswariah	1966	—	—	17 Chlordiazepoxide	—	—	Limited data from postal survey
Facey et al.	1966	59	—	Chlordiazepoxide	—	—	Limited data
Bartholomew and Reynolds	1967	30	M	Chlordiazepoxide	200mg	—	Many other drugs too
Koutsky and Larson	1967	—	—	3 Chlordiazepoxide / 1 Diazepam	—	—	Other drugs and alcohol; limited data
Ewing and Bakewell	1967	—	—	10 Chlordiazepoxide	—	—	Other drugs and alcohol; limited data
Cerny and Cerna	1967	—	—	3 Diazepam	—	—	—
Gordon	1967	40	M	Diazepam	120mg	2 years	Alcohol
		23	F	Diazepam	60mg	1 year	—
Ledda	1968	37	M	Chlordiazepoxide	100mg	2 years	Other drugs too
Säker	1968	41	F	Diazepam	—	—	Other drugs too
Kielholz	1968	—	—	7 Chlordiazepoxide	—	—	General survey with limited information
				15 Diazepam	—	—	May include three cases published separately
Keup	1968	21	F	1 Chlordiazepoxide	—	—	Limited data
Rümmele	1968	—	—	Diazepam	—	—	Alcohol too; limited data
Lunde and Ropsted	1969/1970	—	—	9 Chlordiazepoxide	Av. 85mg	Av. 3 years	Other drugs 3; alcohol 6
				25 Diazepam	Av. 85mg	Av. 2 years	Other drugs 7; alcohol 8
Rickels and Brand	1969	—	—	2 Chlordiazepoxide	—	—	Other drugs; limited data
Holmberg	1969	—	—	1 Chlordiazepoxide	—	—	Some on other drugs; limited evidence on individual cases
				33 Diazepam			
Grant	1969	—	—	1 Diazepam	—	—	Little evidence
Yoshioka et al.	1970	38	M	1 Chlordiazepoxide	—	—	Multiple drugs
Eichner and Aebi	1970	18-22	M	6 Chlordiazepoxide	—	—	Limited data; other drugs and alcohol too
Morse	1970	—	—	1 Chlordiazepoxide	—	—	Limited data; alcohol too
Vaag	1970	35	F	1 Diazepam	—	—	Other drugs
Noble	1970	—	M	1 Chlordiazepoxide	—	—	Limited data; other drugs
Bätig	1970	—	—	18 Chlordiazepoxide	—	—	Very limited data; other drugs and alcohol
				27 Diazepam			
Kryspin-Exner	1970	—	—	1 Chlordiazepoxide	—	—	Limited data; other drugs and alcohol? overlap with 1966 paper
				5 Diazepam			

Authors	Year of publication	Age	Sex	Substance	Benzodiazepine daily dose	Duration	Comments
Worm and Schou	1970	27	M	Chlordiazepoxide	—	—	Limited data; other drugs and alcohol
		37	M	Diazepam	—	—	
		20	M	Chlordiazepoxide	—	—	
Remschmidt and Dauner	1970a,b	15	F	Chlordiazepoxide	—	—	Other drugs and alcohol
		17	M	Diazepam	—	—	Other drugs
Peters and Boeters	1970	23	F	1 Diazepam	70–90mg	1 year	—
		23	F	1 Diazepam	140mg	—	Other drugs
		31	F	1 Diazepam	80mg	2 years	Other drugs
		30	M	1 Diazepam	30mg	3 years	—
		28	M	1 Diazepam	50mg	—	Alcohol
		28	F	1 Diazepam	60–100mg	4 years	Alcohol
		34	F	1 Diazepam	60mg	1 year	Other drugs
Clare	1971	39	F	Diazepam	500mg	Months	Other drugs and alcohol
Weizel	1971	17–22	M	8 Diazepam	—	—	Other drugs; limited data
Runge et al.	1971	—	M	1 Diazepam	—	—	Other drugs
Le Fevre	1971	—	2F	2 Chlordiazepoxide	—	—	Limited data; other drugs and alcohol
				1 Diazepam			
Chambers and Taylor	1971	—	M / F	Chlordiazepoxide and Diazepam	—	—	Multiple drugs
Levy et al.	1092	23	M	Diazepam	—	—	Limited data; other drugs
Nurco and Lerner	1972	—	—	1 Chlordiazepoxide	—	—	No details
				1 Diazepam			
Malcolm	1972	52	F	Diazepam	—	—	Multiple drugs
Petzold	1972	—	F	Diazepam	120mg	1 year	Alcohol
Hoover	1972	—	—	2 Chlordiazepoxide	—	—	Limited data; other drugs
				4 Diazepam			
Reeve	1972	—	—	2 Chlordiazepoxide	—	—	Limited data
				5 Diazepam			Limited data
Mayfield and Montgomery	1972	47	M	1 Chlordiazepoxide	—	—	Limited data; other drugs
Beil	1972	—	M	1 Diazepam	—	—	Limited data; other drugs
Rechenberger	1972	—		5 Diazepam	20–60mg	2–10 years	Limited data
Feuerlein and Busch	1972	—	4F 2M	6 Diazepam	Up to 30mg	2–10 years	Limited data; multiple drugs and alcohol
Darcy	1972	51	M	Nitrazepam	20mg	years	—
Hanna	1972	29	M	Oxazepam	120mg	1¼ years	—
Quitkin et al.	1972	35	F	Chlordiazepoxide	—	—	Other drugs
Mader	1972	16	M	Diazepam	60mg	1 year	Alcohol

Author	Year	Age	Sex	Drug	Dose	Duration	Comments
Venzlaff	1972	38	F	Diazepam	50–100mg	5 years	Other drugs
		30	F	Diazepam	60–130mg	4 years	Other drugs
Badura	1972	44	M	Diazepam	50mg	1½ years	—
Smith	1972	—	—	Diazepam	—	—	Multiple drugs
De Buck	1973	—	—	Lorazepam	10mg	3 weeks	Other drugs
		—	—	Lorazepam	7.5mg	—	—
Swanson et al.	1973	—	—	17 Chlordiazepoxide / 22 Diazepam	—	—	Multiple other drugs including flurazepam; alcohol
Sturner and Garriott	1973	43	F	1 Chlordiazepoxide / 1 Diazepam	—	—	Limited data; other drugs
Ladewig	1973	—	—	1 Chlordiazepoxide / 47 Diazepam	—	—	Limited data; other drugs including nitrazepam; figure adjusted to exclude cases reported previously in Keilholz, 1968
Anonymous	1973	—	—	1 Diazepam	—	—	Limited data; alcohol
Brzezinska and Walczak	1973	14	M	1 Chlordiazepoxide	—	—	Limited data
Morgan et al.	1973	22	F	Diazepam	150mg	—	—
Wätzig and Michaelis	1973	51	M	Diazepam	15mg	7 years	—
Maletzky	1974	20	F	Lorazepam	—	—	Limited data
		27	F	Diazepam	—	—	—
Nerenz	1974	34	M	Diazepam	Up to 100mg	5 years	Limited data
Kellett	1974	—	—	3 Diazepam	50+mg	'months'	Limited data; other drugs
Kawai	1974	43	F	1 Chlordiazepoxide	—	—	Limited data; other drugs
Miller	1974	—	—	1 Chlordiazepoxide	—	—	Limited data
Pearson et al.	1974	—	—	1 Diazepam	—	—	Limited data; multiple drugs
		—	—	1 Diazepam	—	—	—
Hayashki et al.	1974	—	—	3 Diazepam	80+mg	1 month	—
Clift	1975	51	F	Oxazepam	?	2 years	Only limited data: refers to 97 patients psychol. depend
Sjo et al.	1975	—	—	4 Clonazepam	4.75–12mg	11–225 days	Limited data
Vaag	1975	23	M	Diazepam	++	39 days	Very limited data
Sardemann and Friis-Hansen	1975	—	F	3 Diazepam / 1 Mixed	—	—	No details
Anonymous	1975	45	F	Diazepam+Nitrazepam	10mg	—	—
		37	M	Nitrazepam	—	4 years	Other drugs

Authors	Year of publication	Age	Sex	Substance	Benzodiazepine daily dose	Duration	Comments
Malatinsky et al.	1975	66	M	Diazepam	—	—	—
		60	M	Diazepam	—	—	—
Bant	1975	—	F	Diazepam	30mg	1 year	Limited data
		—	F	Diazepam	30mg	2 years	—
Raskind and Bradford	1975	—	—	7 Diazepam	—	'months'	Limited data
Fruensgaard and Vaag	1975	55	F	Nitrazepam	15mg	1½ years	Alcohol
Kellermann	1975	19	M	Diazepam	Up to 200mg	—	Other drugs and alcohol
Misra	1975	33	—	Diazepam	—	—	Multiple drugs including diazepam and chlordiazepoxide
		55	F	Nitrazepam	40-50mg	4 years	
Woody et al.	1975	26	M	Diazepam	150mg	3 weeks	Other drugs
		25	M	Diazepam	15mg	2 weeks	Other drugs
Vyas and Carney	1975	—	F	Diazepam	30mg	3 years	Limited data
Karksgaard	1976	53	F	Lorazepam	1.25-12.5mg	?	
Floyd and Murphy	1976	47-64	2F 3M	5 Diazepam	15-40mg	Months or years	
Beil and Trojan	1976	—	—	Diazepam	—		Limited data; other drugs
Sandman	1976	36	F	1 Diazepam	—		Limited data; alcohol
Fruensgaard	1976	47	F	Diazepam	20-30mg	6-7 years	1 case omitted, see Fruensgaard et al., 1975
		46	F	Diazepam } Nitrazepam	30mg } 5mg	5-6 years	
		49	F	Diazepam } Chlordiazepoxide	30mg } 5mg	'months'	
Rifkin et al.	1976	25	M	Diazepam	30mg	3 months	—
Zisook and De Vaul	1977	34	F	Diazepam	40-60mg	10 years	—
Sumiyoshi and Tsuzuki	1977	46	M	Nitrazepam	10-25mg	3 years	Drugs–no details
Tait and Hutchinson	1977	50	F	1 Mixed	—	—	All with other drugs – no details
Boeszoermenyi and Solti	1977	—		9 Diazepam	—	—	details
Gossop and Roy	1977	—		4 Diazepam	—	—	All with other drugs – no details
Yamasaki et al.	1977	33	M	Diazepam	40-280mg	3 years	
		56	M	Diazepam } Flurazepam	70-100mg } 90-150mg	1½-2 years	
Preskorn and Denner	1977		M	Diazepam	60-80mg	6-8 months	Other drugs
			F	Diazepam	100-160mg	1½ years	

	Year	Age	Sex	Drug	Dose	Duration	
Dysken and Chan	1977	—	M	Diazepam	15–30 mg	7 years	—
Pevnick et al.	1978	37	M	Diazepam	30–45 mg	20 months	+Drugs
Mendelson	1978	24	M	Oxazepam	45 mg	2 years	—
Barry and Weintraub	1978	28	F	Diazepam	100 mg	4 days	+Drugs
Ebihara and Ikeda	1978	55	M	Chlordiazepoxide	150–300 mg	1¼ years	+Drugs
Aligulander and Borg	1978	30	F	Clorazepate	60 mg	Several years	+Drugs
Agrawal	1978	30	F	Diazepam	20–340 mg	5 months	Alcohol
Fox	1978	42	M	Lorazepam	—	—	Limited data
Brown et al.	1978	—	—	3 Chlordiazepoxide	30–100 mg	9-58 months	Other drugs
Minter and Murray	1978	30	M	Diazepam	20–200 mg	Several years	
O'Brien	1978	35	F	Diazepam	30–40 mg	—	Other drugs
Martin et al.	1979	—	—	2 Diazepam / 1 Oxazepam	—	—	Other drugs – no details
Maruta et al.	1979	—	F	4 Diazepam	—	—	Other drugs
Bliding	1979	—	F	Oxazepam	200 mg	8 years	Alcohol
		—	F	Oxazepam	60–90 mg	5 years	—
		—	F	Oxazepam	200–250 mg	—	—
Acuda and Muhangi	1979	30	M	Oxazepam	100 mg	6 months	—
		24	M	Diazepam	10–45 mg	2 years	—
		22	F	Diazepam	5–80 mg	2 years	—
		27	M	Diazepam	150–200 mg	6 months	—
		48	F	Diazepam	5–80 mg	2 years	—
Smith	1979	37	M	Diazepam	10 mg	5 years	+Drugs – 4 other cases suggest overdose psychosis
Teo et al.	1979	29	M	Flunitrazepam	4 mg	'months'	No details
Shinfuku	1979	65	M	Nitrazepam	5 mg	5 years	Paper refers to 10 patients with multiple drug abuse
Tennant	1979	64	F	Diazepam	20–80 mg	4 years	Other drugs
Tagaya and Koshino	1979	27	F	Nitrazepam	60 mg	3 months	Other drugs
		41	M	Nitrazepam	20–50 mg	4 years	Alcohol
		32	F	Nitrazepam	10–15 mg	1 year	—
		36	M	Nitrazepam	30 mg	5 years	Other drugs
Sironi et al.	1979	28	M	Clonazepam	3 mg	1 year	Other drugs
		27	F	Clonazepam	6 mg	1 year	Other drugs
Moerck and Magelund	1979	55	M	Diazepam	80–140 mg	—	—
Miller and Nulsen	1979	37	F	Diazepam	60–80 mg	8 years	—
Laux	1979	26	F	Bromazepam	6–48 mg	3 months	—
Endo and Kubota	1979	76	M	Nitrazepam	5 mg	1 year	—

Authors	Year of publication	Age	Sex	Substance	Benzodiazepine daily dose	Duration	Comments
De Bard	1979	56	M	Diazepam	80mg	4–5 years	Other drugs
Brody	1979	—	M	Flunitrazepam	—	—	—
Tennant	1979	—	—	10 Diazepam 1 Chlordiazepoxide	—	—	Large study of drug abuse
Cohen et al.	1980	24	F	Diazepam	—	8 years	—
Howe	1980	27	F	Lorazepam	7.5mg	4 years	—
De la Fuente et al.	1980	38	F	Lorazepam	8mg	6 months	—
		39	F	Lorazepam	8mg	5 months	—
Einarson	1980	—	M	Lorazepam	12mg	Several months	2 further cases (1 clorazepate, 1 oxazepam) – no details
Chandara	1980	—	F	Lorazepam	4–12mg	2 months	Other drugs
Bismuth et al.	1980	63	M	Diazepam	30mg	8 years	
		63	F	Mixed	—	5 years+	Other drugs
		76	F	Oxazepam/Nitrazepam	—	5 years+	Other drugs
		52	F	Lorazepam/Diazepam	—	5 years+	Other drugs
		34	F	Diazepam	—	5 years	Other drugs
		28	M	Lorazepam	—	6 months	Other drugs
		21	M	Diazepam/Clorazepate	—	1 year	Other drugs
Tyrer et al.	1980	60	F	Nitrazepam/Lorazepam	5mg/7.5mg	6 weeks	
Stewart	1980	51	F	Diazepam	Up to 75mg	4 years	Other drugs
Imoto	1980	—	—	Lorazepam	1mg	—	Limited data
Epstein	1980	60	F	Diazepam	5mg	—	Other drugs
Benzer and Cushman	1980	—	—	25 patients (19 Diazepam 4 Chlordiazepoxide 1 Lorazepam 1 Clorazepate)	15 high dose, 10 normal	0.5–15 years	All patients showed dependence to both alcohol and benzodiazepines
Winokur et al.	1980	32	M	Diazepam	15–25mg	6 years	Diazepam
Tyrer	1980	—	—	Lorazepam	5–15mg	2 years	Other drugs
Khan et al.	1980	38	M	Lorazepam	7.5mg	1 month	Other drugs plus alcohol
		58	F	Lorazepam	10mg	6 months	
		61	M	Oxazepam	60mg	8 years	
		29	F	Lorazepam	7.5mg	3 years	
		32	F	Oxazepam	90mg	3 years	
		35	F	Diazepam	15mg	10 years	
		39	F	Diazepam	15mg	10 years	
		21	F	Lorazepam	4mg	3 years	

122

Author	Year	Age	Sex	Drug	Dose	Duration	Comments
		72	F	Nitrazepam / Oxazepam	10 mg / 50–150 mg	2 years	
		52	F	Nitrazepam / Lorazepam	10 mg / 7.5 mg	15 years	
		28	M	Diazepam / Nitrazepam	60 mg / 10 mg	6 months	
				Lorazepam / Nitrazepam	7.5 mg / 10 mg		
Cushman and Benzer	1980	?		54 Various Benzodiazepines	—	—	See Appendix 2 for details
Petursson and Lader	1981b	36	M	Clobazam	20–30 mg	1 year	Other benzodiazepines for 2½ years
		58	M	Clobazam	30 mg	6 months	Other benzodiazepines for 6 months
Nagy et al.	1981	60	F	Diazepam	100 mg	2 months	A very doubtful case
Schopf	1981	43	F	Flunitrazepam	2–4 mg	3½ years	Schopf (1981) refers to 11 out of 17 patients with dependence but no details given
		50	F	Mixed	—	2½ years	
		51	F	Nitrazepam	5–7.5 mg	13 years	
		42	F	Lorazepam	4–5 mg	7 years	
		39	M	Flurazepam	30 mg	20 days	
		28	M	Mixed	—	4 years	Drugs plus
Boning	1981	39	—	Bromazepam	6–30 mg	18 months	—
		36	—	Bromazepam	12–24 mg	18 months	Other drugs
Walters and Nel	1981	—	—	15 Oxazepam, 15 Chlordiazepoxide	—	—	No further details
Schuster and Humphries	1981	62	M	Diazepam	—	Years	Alcohol
		32	M	Mixed	—	2 years	Alcohol
		41	M	Mixed	—	5 years	Alcohol
Yamashito	1981	45	F	Nitrazepam	100 mg	3 years	—
		46	M	Nitrazepam	10–25 mg	3 months	Plus drugs
		27	F	Nitrazepam	60 mg	4 years	Alcohol
		41	M	Nitrazepam	20–50 mg	1 year	—
		32	F	Nitrazepam	10–15 mg	5 years	Drugs plus
		36	M	Nitrazepam	30 mg	1 year	—
		76	M	Nitrazepam	5 mg	6 months	—
		34	M	Chlordiazepoxide	60–70 mg	—	—
		35	F	Chlordiazepoxide	100–200 mg	1 month	Plus drugs
		37	F	Chlordiazepoxide	150 mg	6 months	Plus drugs
		35	M	Chlordiazepoxide	100–200 mg	2 years	Plus drugs
		29	M	Chlordiazepoxide	200 mg	2 years	Plus drugs
		40	M	Chlordiazepoxide	200–400 mg	1½ years	Plus drugs
		55	M	Chlordiazepoxide	150–300 mg		Plus drugs

Authors	Year of publication	Age	Sex	Substance	Benzodiazepine daily dose	Duration	Comments
Tyrer et al.	1981	—	—	Lorazepam	6 mg	27 months	—
		—	—	Lorazepam	2 mg	6 months	—
		—	—	Lorazepam	3 mg	16 months	—
		—	—	Lorazepam	7.5 mg	2 years	—
		—	—	Diazepam	7.5 mg	10 years	—
		—	—	Diazepam	10 mg	6 years	—
		—	—	Diazepam	5 mg	7 months	—
		—	—	Diazepam	15 mg	10 years	—
		—	—	Diazepam	15 mg	3 years	—
		—	—	Diazepam	15 mg	17 months	—
		—	—	Diazepam	5 mg	2½ years	—
		—	—	Diazepam	5 mg	8 months	—
		—	—	Diazepam	120 mg	7 months	—
		—	—	Diazepam	4 mg	13 years	—
		—	—	Diazepam	6 mg	33 months	—
		—	—	Diazepam	15 mg	11 years	—
		—	—	Diazepam	7.5 mg	6 months	Plus drugs
		—	—	Diazepam	12.5 mg	6 months	—
Ratna	1981	22	M	Temazepam	Up to 100 mg	2 years	Alcohol
Petursson and Lader	1981a	—	9M 7F	10 Diazepam 4 Lorazepam 2 Clobazam	10–30 mg 1.0–7.5 mg 30 mg	1–16 years	
Barton	1981	63	M	Lorazepam	6 mg	41 days	
		63	M	Lorazepam	2 mg	68 days	
Winokur and Rickels	1981	32	M	Diazepam	20 mg	14 weeks	Previous diazepam treatment
Abernethy et al.	1981	31	F	Diazepam	100–200 mg	2 years +	
Haslerud and Heskestad	1981	40	F	Flunitrazepam +Neuroleptic	4–6 mg	2 years	
		53	F	Flunitrazepam	10 mg	?	
				Flunitrazepam	8–12 mg	1 year	
		27	F	Flunitrazepam	9–12 mg	1 year	
		53		Flunitrazepam	2 mg		
Hartviksen	1981	50	M	Nitrazepam	125–150 mg	1 year+	Alcohol
		60	M	Diazepam	50–70 mg	1 year+	Alcohol
Loveridge	1981	36	M	Diazepam	15–60 mg	3 years+	Alcohol
		65	F	Diazepam	5 mg	11 years	Alcohol

Author	Year	Age	Sex	Drug	Dose	Duration	Alcohol
				Diazepam	15 mg	6 years	
Mellor and Jain	1982	67	M	Diazepam	10–15 mg	5 years	Stresses later symptoms +alcohol previously +imipramine (convulsions)
Good and Dubovsky	1982	27	F	Diazepam	Up to 25 mg	3 years	
Simon	1982	39	F	Diazepam	5 mg	3 years	
		30	F	10 Diazepam	60–120 mg	3–14 years	
		31–54	7M	Diazepam+sedative	?	3 years+	
		60	F	Clorazepate	40 mg	4 weeks	
		25	F				
Lennane	1982a	31	F	Oxazepam +glutethimide +chloral hydrate	600 mg	?	Dobbie (1982), Grigor and Dinnen (1982) stress at high doses and multiple therapy make causation unclear, commenting on this paper
		59	F	Oxazepam +amylobarbitone	600 mg	?	
		42	F	Oxazepam +amylobarbitone and fenfluramine	120 mg	?	
Lennane	1982b	50	F	Oxazepam	90 mg	?	
		27	M	Oxazepam	1500 mg	?	
Moore	1982	60+	F	Oxazepam	480–540 mg	4–5 years	Out of 19 benzodiazepine withdrawal cases (17 diazepam; 1 oxazepam; 1 flurazepam). Second case alcohol+other drugs
Robinson and Sellers	1982	28	F	Diazepam	50–100 mg	6 years	
		22	F	Diazepam	120–200 mg	20 months	
		27	M	Diazepam	100–150 mg	12 years	
Holt and Perez-Cruet	1982	25	M	Diazepam	100 mg	5 years	+other drugs
Berlin and Conell	1983	37	M	Flurazepam	30 mg	8 years	On substitution of temazepam
Woimant et al.	1983	42	F	Flunitrazepam	2 mg	12 years	+Maprotiline
Hayner and Inaba	1983	30	M	Lorazepam	6–10 mg	1 year	+Diazepam and flunitrazepam
		41	F	Diazepam	10–15 mg	months	+other sedatives
Leung and Guze	1983	40	F	Diazepam	5–15 mg	7 years	+Imipramine (convulsions)
Ananth	1983	31	M	Oxazepam	45–90 mg	1 year	
Wilbur and Kulik	1983			Diazepam			
Fontaine et al.	1984	19–58		Bromazepam	Not detailed	Not detailed	Paper ascribes changes to rebound anxiety but proportion show withdrawal effects; demonstrates difficulty of interpretation

125

Authors	Year of publication	Age	Sex	Substance	Benzodiazepine daily dose	Duration	Comments
Winokur and Rickels	1984	38	F	Clorazepate	22.5 mg	5 years	
		39	F	Clorazepate	22.5 mg	18 months	Barbiturates
Coid	1984	54	F	Diazepam	20 mg	20 years+	+Other psychotropics
Kahan and Haskett	1984	81	F	Lorazepam	1–2 mg		
Levy	1984	77	M	Alprazolam	5 mg	3 months	After flurazepam 60 mg daily for 10 years+
Berezak et al.	1984	43	M	Triazolam	5 mg	4 years	+Bromazepam, diazepam and alcohol
Edwards and Glen-Bott	1984	50	M	Diazepam	15–30 mg		Both had epileptiform attacks after discontinuing benzodiazepines and receiving epileptogenic viloxazine
				Chlordiazepoxide	30 mg		
				Nitrazepam	5–10 mg		
		32	F	Lorazepam	6 mg		
Fleming	1984	28	M	Triazolam	5.0–7.5 mg	?	+Alcohol, diazepam and multiple drugs
Petursson and Lader	1984	30	F	Diazepam	15–90 mg	11 years	+Nitrazepam and chlordiazepoxide
		39	M	Diazepam	30–200 mg	10 years	+Alcohol and barbiturates
		34	M	Diazepam	15 mg	1 year	
		39	M	Diazepam	20 mg	10 years	+Alcohol and barbiturates
		36	M	Clobazam	30 mg	2 years	+Alcohol
		40	F	Lorazepam	Up to 7.5 mg	2 years	
		33	M	Diazepam	12–40 mg	13 years	
		42	F	Lorazepam	1–7.5 mg	2 years	+Nitrazepam
		62	F	Diazepam	10–20 mg	12 years	+Barbiturates
		35	M	Diazepam	20 mg	12 years	
		31	F	Diazepam	15 mg	11 years	+Illicit drugs
		28	F	Diazepam	2–20 mg	2 years	+Nitrazepam
		30	F	Diazepam	15–90 mg	11 years	+Nitrazepam and chlordiazepoxide
		39	M	Diazepam	30–200 mg	10 years	+Alcohol and barbiturates
		34	M	Diazepam	15 mg	1 year	
		39	M	Diazepam	20 mg	10 years	+Alcohol and barbiturates
		36	M	Clobazam	30 mg	2 years	+Alcohol
		40	F	Lorazepam	Up to 7.5 mg	2 years	
		33	M	Diazepam	12–40 mg	13 years	
		42	F	Lorazepam	1–7.5 mg	2 years	+Nitrazepam

Study	Age	Sex	Drug	Dosage	Duration	Comments
	62	F	Diazepam	10–20 mg	12 years	+Barbiturates
	35	M	Diazepam	20 mg	12 years	+Illicit drugs
	31	F	Diazepam	15 mg	11 years	+Nitrazepam
	28	F	Diazepam	2–20 mg	2 years	
	32	M	Diazepam	15 mg	4 years	
	34	M	Diazepam	7.5 mg	12 years	
	47	F	Lorazepam	60 mg	2 years	
	56	F	Diazepam	15 mg	5 years	
	31	F	Lorazepam	1 mg	2 years	Earlier diazepam
	33	F	Lorazepam	5 mg	5 years	+Alcohol
	48	M	Lorazepam	5 mg	15 years	+Alcohol, previous diazepam
	43	M	Diazepam	15 mg	10 years	
	58	M	Clobazam	30 mg	12 years	
	49	F	Nitrazepam	5 mg	9 years	Previous chlordiazepoxide 5 years
	32	M	Oxazepam	90 mg	6 years	+Alcohol and illicit drugs
	22	M	Diazepam	7.5 mg	2 years	Previous diazepam 1 year
	58	M	Diazepam	10 mg	15 years	+Alcohol
	29	M	Diazepam	30 mg	6 years	
	22	M	Lorazepam	2 mg	2 years	Previous diazepam 12 years
	36	F	Diazepam	30 mg	5 years	+Alcohol and illicit drugs
	36	F	Diazepam	30 mg+	3 years	+lorazepam 1 mg
	37	M	Clobazam	60 mg	2 years	
	32	M	Diazepam	15 mg	9 years	
	50	M	Diazepam	10 mg	7 years	
	49	F	Diazepam	20 mg	12 years	+triazolam 0.125 mg
	70	F	Lorazepam	2.5 mg	6 years	
	37	F	Lorazepam	2 mg	12 years	Previous diazepam 11 years
	49	F	Diazepam	10 mg	7 years	+Illicit drugs
	49	F	Lorazepam	3 mg	1 year	
	27	M	Nitrazepam	30 mg	6 years	—
Breier et al. 1984	35	M	Alprazolam	8 mg	4 months	Seizure on chlorpromazine
Sironi et al. 1984	19	F	Alprazolam	4 mg	4½ months	+Phenobarbital and carbamazepine
	37	F	Clonazepam	3–6 mg		+Phenobarbital
	38	F	Clonazepam	3–6 mg		+Carbamazepine
	28	M	Clonazepam	3–6 mg		
Bond and Schwartz 1984	60	F	Flurazepam	30 mg	9 months	
	52	M	Flurazepam	30–150 mg	6 years	+Sedatives

Appendix 2
Studies on the incidence of withdrawal reactions with benzodiazepines at therapeutic dosage

The following studies provide information (often conflicting information, some qualitative, some quantitative) on the incidence of withdrawal reactions in those taking long-term continuous benzodiazepines at *therapeutic* dosage levels.

The nature of the withdrawal reaction is often not clearly defined. Sometimes it appears that it is a mild and short-lived rebound anxiety or insomnia; sometimes the time sequence suggests a return of the anxiety for which treatment was required; sometimes it is a true abstinence syndrome of alcohol-sedative type.

There are few, if indeed any, of these studies in which the design cannot be criticised.

(a) Few are double-blind controlled; normally the physician is at least aware at what stage dose reduction or removal is to take place.

(b) In some the cut-off is not absolute at a specific time but a form of dose reduction precedes the withdrawal.

(c) The patient has frequently been told about the discontinuation, and with recent media coverage may be anticipating problems (pseudo withdrawal reactions).

(d) With the ready availability of benzodiazepines, withdrawal cannot be assumed unless blood determinations demonstrate falling levels, but such procedures alert the patient to alterations in therapy.

(e) In several of the studies that have been extensively quoted as determining an incidence, the patients have clearly been selected on the basis that they have experienced prior difficulty in stopping.

(f) In very few studies has there been a comparison of pre-treatment

128

against post-withdrawal complaints, yet most reports attribute all post-withdrawal manifestations to the abstinence syndrome.

(g) Despite the observation that many of the symptoms are experienced by 'normal' people this background 'noise' factor is hardly ever considered.

(h) It is usually far from clear whether the complaints were volunteered or prompted by a structured questionnaire.

(i) *Some at least* of the patients must be regarded as having a neurotic personality and being high complainants.

(j) Previous history of barbiturate use, which is known to affect the picture, is often not excluded.

(k) Some of the patients appear to be multiple drug users or alcohol takers but are not excluded.

Despite all these possible criticisms it is important to *try* to determine the risk of withdrawal effects and the studies reported here are the only ones that even make such an attempt.

Each of these studies is mentioned briefly even if I do not believe that they provide relevant information. Others may judge the validity of these studies.

1. Hollister *et al.* (1961)
   This study, which was the first to demonstrate withdrawal, was conducted with doses that were substantially above the therapeutic level and are, according to the author himself, not relevant.

2. Covi *et al.* (1969, 1973)
   45 mg/day chlordiazepoxide was given daily to anxious neurotic patients. Abrupt discontinuation at 10 weeks produced no withdrawal phenomena. After 20 weeks continuous treatment, abrupt discontinuation produced some relatively mild withdrawal effects (though whether withdrawal or return of anxiety is not clear). The situation is complicated by the fact that half the patients were pre-treated with phenobarbitone for 10 weeks.

3. Kryspin-Exner and Demel (1975)
   Kryspin-Exner and Demel found four dependent patients in a group of 111 alcoholics treated for prolonged periods with chlordiazepoxide, and seven among 302 similarly treated with diazepam. Of the 11 who became dependent on benzodiazepines seven were already dependent on other drugs, i.e. representing a benzodiazepine dependence incidence between 1% and 3%.

4. Clift (1975)
   In 50 patients with insomnia treated with diazepam or nitrazepam for 4 years, approximately 15–20% showed evidence of dependence.

5. Maletzky and Klotter (1976)

These authors interviewed 50 subjects who had received a mean daily dose of 16 mg diazepam for an average of 26 months. Assessors felt that of the 24 patients who had tried to discontinue 70% showed some withdrawal effects, but only eight of these patients rated themselves as moderately or severely dependent.

6. Rothstein et al. (1976)

Rothstein et al., in 108 patients with alcoholism who received benzodiazepines (mainly chlordiazepoxide) for over a year, found 5% with evidence of clinical dependence. Yet in this group a higher than average result would be anticipated.

7. Marks (1978)

Marks attempted to assess the incidence of dependence on the basis of published reports. These calculations, though widely quoted, have not subsequently been shown to be wrong. The fault in the study is that while it records *published* cases (whether in the medical press or to health authorities), it cannot determine the proportion of overall cases that are published, i.e. the true incidence in practice.

8. Tyrer et al. (1980, 1981, 1983)

This study, in Nottingham, is one of the few which has attempted to determine the incidence of physical dependence by placebo (or propanolol) substitution. Eighty-six patients were eligible to enter the trial on the basis of at least 4 months regular benzodiazepine use. Forty agreed to take part. Of these, 45% experienced two or more 'withdrawal symptoms' during the 14th day of the study, while 27% showed the typical peak of withdrawal symptoms.

It is important to appreciate that though entry to the study required only 4 months previous use, the majority of those experiencing withdrawal reactions had received therapy for several years (average about 4 years). Hence the high percentage applies to those who have received continuous therapy for several years.

In a recent study by the same group (Tyrer et al., 1983) 22% of patients experienced withdrawal symptoms at a time when they thought their drugs were being withdrawn but the dosage had remained constant, demonstrating the current extent of pseudo withdrawal.

9. Cushman and Benzer (1980)

This was an inpatient study of drug abusers. Sixty-nine of these patients showed urinary evidence of benzodiazepine intake (54 without evidence of other psychoactive drugs in the urine). Of these only one used benzodiazepines alone, 38 with alcohol and 15 with multiple drugs.

For the high-dose benzodiazepine–alcohol abusers the incidence of withdrawal reactions was about 50%. Among the 'low-dose' group (41 patients) none showed a significant withdrawal reaction.

130

10. Murray (1981)

On the basis of a postal questionnaire survey of 183 present users and 78 past users, most of whom had used psychotropic drugs for over 5 years, Murray reported a high proportion who claimed they would find it difficult or impossible to do without psychotropic drugs. The study did not distinguish between dependence or therapeutic need, and—the selection method would encourage replies by those with difficulties.

11. Petursson and Lader (various reports 1981–1984)

The Petursson and Lader studies have been quoted fairly frequently as evidence of a high incidence of dependence. These excellent studies of the dependence phenomenon do not provide valid evidence of the practical incidence of withdrawal problems because they were based on a selected group who had previously tried to discontinue therapy.

12. Rickels with others (1981, 1982, 1983)

Rickels *et al.* in a prospective study of 129 patients given 15–40 mg diazepam daily (i.e. rather a high daily dose by the standards of many countries) found that after 6 weeks of therapy two showed withdrawal symptoms; but both these had received more than 8 months therapy on a previous occasion and should therefore be discounted. After 14 weeks of therapy there were eight with definite withdrawal symptoms and three with transient symptoms. Of those with definite withdrawal symptoms, four had received more than 8 months previous therapy and a further three were alcohol consumers, i.e. there was only one with definite abstinence symptoms with benzodiazepine alone. Two of the three patients with transient symptoms had received up to 8 months previous therapy. After 22 weeks there were four definite and four transient withdrawals, but three of each had received more than 8 months previous therapy, i.e. there was again only one definite withdrawal reaction.

If the situation is considered of those who had at least 8 months previous treatment (most well over a year) 43% showed definite and 14% transient reactions. This can be compared with 2% definite withdrawal and 4% transient reactions under 8 months continuous use if those consuming alcohol are excluded.

13. Marks (1981)

Marks undertook a small controlled study of abrupt withdrawal in a group of patients who had received diazepam 10 mg or 15 mg continuously for over a year. Substitution was with either placebo or the same dose of diazepam presented in exactly the same form as the placebo but unlike normal diazepam.

The trial was discontinued after 27 patients (12 diazepam and 15 placebo substitution) because it was very difficult to find patients in the Cambridge area who were on *continuous* diazepam at that dosage and because just criticism was made that without blood level determination the possibility of use of hoarded diazepam could not be excluded. Of the 15 in the withdrawal group only one patient experienced withdrawal effects (after 4 years at 10 mg/day regularly).

14. Ladewig *et al.* (1981)

    This was a survey of 7428 practising Swiss physicians, of whom 72.9% replied. From this survey 180 patients with isolated benzodiazepine abuse (i.e. mainly dependence during therapeutic use) were identified and confirmed. Fifty-five of these 180 patients had not experienced withdrawal symptoms and cannot validly be termed physically dependent. However, on the basis of the full 180 patients Ladewig *et al.* calculate that this corresponds to only two abuse patients per 100000 prescriptions. The majority were very long-term users.

15. Hallstrom and Lader (1981)

    Hallstrom and Lader, on the basis of a postal survey of 71 phobic patients who had received long-term benzodiazepines (mainly for over 4 years), suggested that some 25% showed two or more symptoms that are regarded as indicating withdrawal reactions.

16. Laughren *et al.* (1982)

    In a study of 24 patients who had received diazepam at a mean dose of 17 mg/day for a mean duration of 5 years (range 1–12 years) there was no clear evidence of withdrawal reactions.

17. Ashton (1984)

    The recent report by Ashton (1984) has also been taken as evidence of a substantial incidence of dependence, but it is a report of individual selected patients and not a prospective study to determine incidence.

18. Fontaine *et al.* (1984)

    This was a double-blind placebo-controlled trial of 4 weeks of benzodiazepines (bromazepam 18 mg/day or diazepam 15 mg/day) followed by 3 weeks abrupt or gradual withdrawal. Abrupt withdrawal produced a significantly greater ($p = <0.05$) level of anxiety-related symptoms which might represent either return of the anxiety or the development of dependence after 4 weeks treatment. The study should be interpreted with caution because only six of the patients had not previously been treated with benzodiazepines. About half had received over 1 year's treatment in the period prior to the trial. The majority therefore represent long-term users.

19. Murphy *et al.* (1984)

    In this study of diazepam (5–20 mg daily) for either 6 or 12 weeks (10 in each group) by the Tyrer group, sudden withdrawal after 6 weeks led to a significant increase in a symptom rating scale. As opposed to this the group which received diazepam for 12 weeks did not show a significant increase on sudden withdrawal. The authors suggest that this indicates pharmacological dependence rather than

132

rebound anxiety after only 6 weeks therapy, since two other groups treated with buspirone showed no similar increase. Since the results show inconsistency they should be regarded with caution until confirmed. The other worry about this study, on the basis of personal experience, is whether they are really all 'virgin anxiety patients', i.e. not having received any prior therapy or high alcohol intake.

References

Abernethy, D. R., Greenblatt, D. J.and Shader, R. I. (1981). Treatment of diazepam withdrawal syndrome with propranolol. *Ann. Int. Med.*, **44,** 354

Abrahamson, A. (1976). Psychotropic drug use: fallacies and a paradox. *Psychol. Med.*, **6,** 529–531

Acuda, S. W. and Muhangi, J. (1979). Diazepam addiction in Kenya. *East Afr. Med. J.*, **56,** 76–79

Addiction Research Foundation (1980). Report of the 'International Working Group on the Convention on Psychotropic Substances, 1971, 8–12 September, Alcohol and Addiction Research Foundation

Agrawal, P. (1978). Diazepam addiction – a case report. *Can. Psychiatr. Assoc. J.*, **23,** 35–37

Aivazian, G. H. (1964). Clinical evaluation of diazepam. *Dis. Nervous Syst.*, **25,** 491–496

Allgulander, C. (1978). Dependence on sedative and hypnotic drugs. A comparative clinical and social study. *Acta Psychiatr. Scand. Suppl.*, **270**

Allgulander, C. and Borg, S. (1978). A delirious abstinence syndrome associated with clorazepate, *Br. J. Addict.*, **73,** 175–177

Allgulander, C., Borg, S. and Vikander, B. (1984). A 4–6 follow-up of 50 patients with primary dependence on sedative and hypnotic drugs. *Am. J. Psychiatr.*, **141,** 1580–1582

Altshuler, H. L. and Phillips, P. E. (1978). Intragastric self-administration of drugs by the primate. In Ho, B. T., Richards III, D. W. and Chute, D. L. (eds.). *Drug Discrimination and State Dependent Learning.* p. 263. (New York: Academic Press)

Amit, Z. and Cohen, J. (1974). The effect of hypothalamic stimulation on oral ingestion of diazepam in rats, *Behav. Biol.*, **10,** 223

Ananth, J. (1983). Abstinence syndrome from therapeutic doses of oxazepam., *Can. J. Psychiatr.*, **28,** 592

Anonymous (1965). Endstation Nervenheilanstalt. *Nat. Zeitung. Basel*, **123,** 6

Anonymous (1973). Diazepam induced hepatitis. *Drug Ther.*, **3,** 88

Anonymous (1975). Information on adverse reactions to drugs, *Jpn. Med. Gaz.*, **12,** 10–11, 13

APA (1980). *Diagnostic and Statistical Manual of Mental Disorders*, Third edition, Washington, DC

Ashton, H. (1984). Benzodiazepine withdrawal: an unfinished story, *Br. Med. J.*, **288,** 1135–1140

Athinarayanan, P., Pierog, S. H., Nigam, S. K. and Glass, L. (1976). Chlordiazepoxide withdrawal in the neonate. *Am. J. Obstet. Gynecol.*, **124,** 212–213

Ator, N. and Griffiths, R. R. (1982). Oral self-administation of triazolam and diazepam in the baboon: effects of benzodiazepine antagonist. ISGIDAR Meeting, Toronto, Canada, 27 June

Ayd, F. J. (1980). Benzodiazepines: social isues: misuse and abuse. *Psychosomatics*, **21**, Supp., 21–25

Ayd, F. (1981). Diazepam – the question of long-term therapy and withdrawal reactions. *Drug Therapy*, Special Supplement

Ayd, F. (1983). Benzodiazepine dependence and withdrawal. *J. Psychoactive Drugs*, **15**, 67–70

Backes, C. R. and Cordero, L. (1980). Withdrawal symptoms in the neonate from presumptive intrauterine exposure to diazepam: report of case. *J. Am. Obstet. Assoc.*, **79**, 584–585

Badura, H. O. (1972). Valiumsucht: Beobachtung zum Thema, Valiumsucht. *Internistische Praxis*, **12**, 349 and 352

Bakewell, W. E. and Wikler, A. (1966). Non-narcotic addiction: incidence in a university hospital psychiatric ward. *J. Am. Med. Assoc.*, **196**, 710–713

Balter, M. B., Levine, J. and Manheimer, D. I. (1974). Cross-national study of the extent of anti-anxiety/sedative drug use. *New Eng. J. Med.*, **290**, 769–774

Balmer, R., Battegay, R., Von Marschall, R. (1981). Long-term treatment with diazepam: investigation of consumption habits and the interaction between psychotherapy and psychopharmacotherapy: a prospective study. *Int. Pharmacopsychiat.*, **16**, 221–234

Balter, M. B., Manheimer, D. I., Mellinger, G. D. and Cisin, I. H. (1983). Cross-national comparisons of anti-anxiety/sedative drug use. Read before the international symposium entitled 'Rational Prescribing of Benzodiazepines', Vienna, 10 July.

Balter, M. B., Manheimer, D. I., Mellinger, G. D. and Uhlenhuth, E. H. (1984). A cross-national comparison of anti-anxiety/sedative drug use. In Rational prescribing of benzodiazepines. *Curr. Med. Res. Opin.* (Suppl. 4), **8**, 5–20

Bant, W. (1975). Diazepam withdrawal symptoms. *Br. Med. J.*, **4**, 295

Bantutova, I., Ovcharov, R. and Koburova, K. (1978). Changes in the convulsion threshold and in the level of brain biogenic amines in rats chronically treated with phenobarbital or diazepam. *Acta Physiol. Pharmacol. Bulgaria*, **4**, 26

Barry, D. J. and Weintraub, M. (1978). Barbiturate management of withdrawal syndromes. *Drug Ther.*, **8**, 83–86

Barten, H. H. (1965). Toxic psychosis with transient dysmnestic syndrome following withdrawal from Valium. *Am. J. Psychiatry*, **121**, 1201–1211

Bartholomew, A. and Reynolds, W. S. (1967). Four cases of progressive drug abuse. *Med. J. Austr.*, **54**, 653–657

Barton, D. F. (1981). More on lorazepam withdrawal. *Drug Intell. Clin. Phar.*, **15**, 134

Bass, M. J. (1981). Do physicians overprescribe for women with emotional problems? *Can. Med. Assoc. J.*, **125**, 1211

Bass, M. J. and Baskerville, J. C. (1981). Prescribing of minor tranquillizers for emotional problems in family practice. *Can. Med. Assoc. J.*, **125**, 1225–1226

Battig, K. (1970). Konsum psychoaktiver und illegaler Drogen bei zurcher hochschulstudenten. *Schweiz. Med. Wschr.*, **100**, 1887

Beil, H. (1972). Rauschmittelmissbrauch aus der Sicht des Arztes fuer Allgeneinmedizin. *Therapiewoche*, **22**, 3733–3745

Beil, H. and Trojan, A. (1976). Tilidin/Valoron-Missbrauch. Ergebnisse einer Befragung von Drogenkonsumenten. *Munch. Med. Wochenschr.*, **118**, 633–638

Belknap, J. K. (1978). Barbiturate physical dependence in mice: effects of neuroleptics and diazepam on the withdrawal syndrome. *Clin. Toxicol.*, **2**, 427

Benzer, D. and Cushman, P. (1980). Alcohol and benzodiazepines: withdrawal syndromes. *Alcoholism: Clin. Exp. Res.*, **4**, 243–247

Berezak, A., Weber, M., Hansmann, J. *et al.* (1984). Dependence physique aux

REFERENCES

benzodiazepines dans un contexte traumatologique. *Ann. Fr. Anesth. Reanim.*, **3,** 383–384

Berlin, R. M. and Connell, C. J. (1983). Withdrawal symptoms after long term treatment with therapeutic doses of flurazepam. *Am. J. Psychiatr.*, **110,** 488–490

Binder, W. Kornhuber, H. H. and Waiblinger, G. (1984). *Benzodiazepin-Sucht, unsere iatrogene Seuche – 157 Faelle von Benzodiazepin-Abhaengigkeit.* Oeff. Gesundh.-Wes. **46,** 80–86 (Stuttgart–New York: Georg Thieme Verlag)

Birmingham (1978). Practice activity analysis.4.Psychotropic drugs – from the Birmingham research unit of the R. Coll. of Gen. Pract., *J. R. Coll. Gen. Pract.*, **28,** 122–124

Bismuth, C., Le Bellec, M., S. and Lagier, G. (1980). Dependence physique aux benzodiazepines. *N. Presse Med.*, **9,** 1941–1945

Blackwell, B. (1973). Psychotropic Drugs in Use Today. The Role of Diazepam in Medical Practice. *J. Am. Med. Assoc.*, **225,** 1637

Blaha, L. and Brueckmann, J. U. (1983). Benzodiazepines in the treatment of anxiety (Angst): European experience. In Costa, E. (ed.). *The Benzodiazepines: from Molecular Biology to Clinical Practice.* pp. 311–324 (New York: Raven Press)

Bliding, A. (1979). The abuse potential of benzodiazepines with special reference to oxazepam. *Acta Psychiatr. Scand. Suppl.*, **274,** 111–116

Blum, K., Eubanks, J. D., Wallace, J. E. and Hamilton, H. (1976). Enhancement of alcohol withdrawal convulsions in mice by haloperidol. *Clin. Toxicol.*, **9,** 427

Boeszoermenyi, Z. and Solti, G. (1977). Ueber Einige atypische Entziehungssyndrome bei Polytoxikomanien. *Pharmatherapeutica*, **1,** 570–572.

Boethius, G. and Westerholm, B. (1976). Is the use of hypnotics, sedatives and minor tranquillizers really a major health problem? *Acta Med. Scand.*, **199,** 507–512

Boisse, N. R., Ikamoto, H. and Michiko, K. (1978). Physical dependence to barbital compared to pentobarbital. I. 'Chronically equivalent' dosing method. *J. Pharmacol. Exp. Ther.*, **204,** 497

Boisse, N. R., Ryan, G. P. and Guarino, J. J. (1982). Experimental induction of benzodiazepine physical dependence in rodents. In *Problems of Drug Dependence, 1982.* Proceedings of 43rd Annual Scientific Meeting, NIDA Monograph, U.S. Printing Office, Washington, **41,** 191

Boisse, N. R., Ryan, G. P., Guarino, J. J. and Gay, M. H. (1981). Comparison of benzodiazepine and barbiturate tolerance and physical dependence in the rat. *Pharmacologist*, **23,** 192

Bond, A. J. and Lader, M. H. (1981). Comparative effects of diazepam and buspirone on subjective feelings, psychological tests and the EEG. *Int. Pharmacopsychiatry*, **16,** 212–220

Bond, W. S. and Schwartz, M. (1984). Withdrawal reactions after long-term treatment with flurazepam. *Clin. Pharmacol.*, **3,** 316–318

Boning, J. (1981). Entzugsdelirien unter Bromazepam (Lexotanil). *Nervenartz*, **52,** 293–297

Bowden, C. L. and Fisher, J. G. (1980). Safety and efficacy of long-term diazepam therapy. *South. Med. J.*, **73,** 1581–1584

Bowes, H. A. (1965). The role of diazepam (Valium) in emotional illness. *Psychosomatics*, **6,** 336–340

Braestrup, C. and Squires, R. F. (1977). Brain specific benzodiazepine receptors in rat characterized by high affinity ^{3}H-diazepam binding. *Proc. Natl. Acad. Sci.*, **74,** 3805–3809

Breier, A., Charney, D. S. and Nelson, J. C. (1984). Seizures induced by abrupt discontinuation of alprazolam. *Am. J. Psychiatry* **141,** 1606–1607

Broadhurst, P. L. (1959). *Acta Psychol.*, **16,** 321

Brody, R. (1979). The story behind the pharmacist who got hooked on Rx Drugs. *Am. Druggist*, **179**, 32–36

Brown, B. S. and Chaitkin, L. (1981). Use of stimulant/depressant drugs by drug abuse clients in selected metropolitan areas. *Int. J. Addict.*, **16**, 1473–1490

Brown, W. A., Laughren, T. P. and Williams, B. W. (1978). Neuroendocrine correlates of clinical response during withdrawal from chlordiazepoxide. *Comm. Psychopharmacol.*, **2**, 251–254

Brzezinska, I. and Walczak, B. (1973). 14 przypadkow toksykomanii wsrod mlodziezy. *Polski tygodnik Lek.*, **28**, 696–697

Budd, R. D. (1981). The use of diazepam and of cocaine in combination with other drugs by Los Angeles county probationers. *Am. J. Drug. Alcohol Abuse*, **8**, 249–255

Burke, G. W. and Anderson, C. W. G. (1962). Response to Librium in individuals with a propensity for addiction: a pilot study. *J. Louisiana State Med. Soc.*, **114**, 58–60

Bush, P. J., Spector, K. K. and Rabin, D. L. (1984). Use of sedatives and hypnotics prescribed in a family practice. *South. Med. J.*, **77**, 677–681

Busto, U., Naranjo, C. A., Cappell, H. *et al.* (1983a). Patterns of benzodiazepine abuse (BA). *Clin. Pharmacol. Ther.*, **33**, 237

Busto, U., Simpkins, J., Sellers, E. M. *et al.* (1983b). Objective determination of benzodiazepine use and abuse in alcoholics. *Br. J. Addict.*, **78**, 429–435

Cahalan, D. and Cisin, I. H. (1968). American drinking practices; summary of findings from a national probability sample 1. Extent of drinking by population subgroups. *Q. J. Study Alcohol*, **29**, 130–151

Cerny, M. and Cerna, H. (1967). Lecba fobii chlordiazepoxidem a diazepamem. *Activ. Nerv. Superior*, **9**, 371

Chait, L. D., Uhlenhuth, E. H. and Johanson, C. E. (1984). An experimental paradigm for studying the discriminative stimulus properties of drugs in humans. *Psychopharmacology*, **82**, 272–274

Chambers, C. D. and Taylor, W. J. R. (1971). Patterns of propoxyphene abuse. *Int. J. Clin. Pharmacol.*, **4**, 240

Chandara, D. B. (1980). Delayed diazepam withdrawal syndrome: a case of auditory and visual hallucinations and seizures. *J. Med. Assoc. Ga.*, **69**, 769–770

Clare, A. W. (1971). Diazepam, alcohol and barbiturate abuse. *Br. Med. J.*, **4**, 340

Clift, A. D. (1975). Sleep disturbance in General Practice. In Clift, A. D. (ed.). *Sleep disturbance and hypnotic drug dependence*. Amsterdam: Excerpta Medica.

Cohen, M. W., Masters, J. S. and Doyle, C. C. (1980). Relaxation-facilitated EMG biofeedback in the treatment of diazepam withdrawal syndrome: a case study. *Am. J. Clin. Biofeedback*, **3**, 68–70

Cohen, S. (1976). Valium: its use and abuse. *Drug Abuse Alc. Newsl.*, **5**, No. 4

Coid, J. (1984). Relief of diazepam–withdrawal syndrome by shoplifting. *Br. J. Psychiatry*, **145**, 552–554

Cole, J. O. *et al.* (1982a). Assessment of the abuse liability of buspirone in recreational sedative users. *J. Clin. Psychiatry*, **43**, 69–74

Cole, J. O., Orzack, M. H., Benes, F. M., Beake, B. J., Bird, M. P. *et al.* (1982b). Subjective effects of benzodiazepines and methaqualone in recreational sedative users. *Psychopharmacol. Bull.*, **18**, No. 3, 87–96

Conell, L. J. and Berlin, R. M. (1983). Withdrawal after substitution of a short-acting for a long-acting benzodiazepine. *J. Am. Med. Assoc.*, **250**, 2838–2840

Consensus Conference (1983). *Drugs and Insomnia: the use of medications to promote sleep*. Nat. Inst. Health. Bethesda, November.

Costa, E., Guidotti, A and Mao, C. C. (1975). Evidence for involvement of GABA in the action of benzodiazepines: studies on rat cerebellum. In Costa, E. and Greengard P. (eds.) *Mechanism of Action of Benzodiazepines*. pp. 113–130. (New York: Raven Press)

REFERENCES

Covi, L., Kipmanir, S., Pattison, J. H. *et al.* (1973). Length of treatment with anxiolytic sedatives and response to their sudden withdrawal. *Acta Psychiatr. Scand.*, **49**, 51-64

Covi, L., Park, L. E., Lipman, R. S., Uhlenhuth, E. H. and Rickels, K. (1969). Factors affecting withdrawal response to certain minor tranquilizers. In Cole J. and Wittenborn, (eds.) *Drug Abuse: Social and Psychopharmacological Aspects.* (Springfield: C. Thomas)

Cumin, R., Bonetti, E. P., Scherschlicht, R. and Haefely, W. E. (1982). Use of the specific benzodiazepine antagonist, Ro 15-1788, in studies of physiological dependence on benzodiazepines. *Experientia (Basel)*, **38**, 833–834

Cushman, P. and Benzer, D. (1980). Benzodiazepines and drug abuse: Clinical observations in chemically dependent persons before and during abstinence. *Drug and Alcohol Dependence*, **6**, 365–371

Czerwenka-Wenkstetten, A., Hofmann, G. and Kryspin-Exner, K. (1965). Ein Fall von Valium-Entzugsdelier. *Wien. Med. Wochenschr.*, **115**, 994–995

Dally, A. (1983). Drug users and urine testing. *Lancet*, **1**, 575

Darcy, L. (1972). Delirium tremens following withdrawal of nitrazepam. *Med. J. Austr.*, **59**, 450

Davies, B., Thorley, A. and O'Connor, D. (1985). Progression of addiction careers in young adult solvent misusers. *Br. Med. J.*, **290**, 109–110

Davis, W. M., Smith, S. G. and Werner, T. E. (1978). Variables influencing chlordiazepoxide self-administration behavior of rats. *Fed. Proc.*, **37**, 828

De Bard, M. L. (1979). Diazepam withdrawal syndrome: a case with psychosis seizure and coma. *Am. J. Psychiatry*, **136**, 104–105

De Buck, R. (1973). Clinical experience with lorazepam in the treatment of neurotic patients. *Curr. Med. Res. Opin.*, **1**, 291–295

De la Fuente, J. R., Rosenbaum, A. H., Martin, H. R. and Niven. R. G. (1980). Lorazepam-related withdrawal seizures. *Mayo Clin. Proc.*, **53**, 190–192

De Wit, H., Johanson, C. E., Uhlenhuth, E. H. and McCrachen, S. (1983). The effects of two non-pharmacological variables on drug preference in humans. In L. S. Harris (ed.). *Problems of Drug Dependence*. Natl. Inst. Drug Abuse Res. Monogr. Ser. 43, US Dept. Health and Human Services, Washington DC/US, 251–257

De Wit, H., and Johanson, C. E. (1983). Preference for lorazepam in humans. *Fed. Proc.*, **42**, 345

De Wit, H., Johanson, C. E. and Uhlenhuth, E. H. (1984a). The dependence potential of benzodiazepines. *Curr. Med. Res. Opin.*, **8**, 48–59

De Wit, H., Uhlenhuth, E. H. and Johanson, C. E. (1984b). Individual differences in drug preference. *Pharmacol. Biochem. Behav.*, **20**, 988

De Wit, H., Uhlenhuth, E. H., Pierri, J. and Johanson, C. E. (1984c). Preference for pentobarbital and diazepam in normal volunteer subjects. *Fed. Proc.*, **43**, 931

Deneau, G. A. (1969). Psychogenic dependence in monkeys. In Steinberg, H. (ed.) *Scientific Basis of Drug Dependence*. p. 199 (London: Churchill)

Deneau, G. A. and Weiss, S. (1968). A substitution technique for determining barbiturate-like physiological dependence capacity in the dog. *Pharmacopsychiat. Neuro-Psychopharmakol.*, **1**, 270

Dennis, P. J. (1979). Monitoring of psychotropic drug prescribing in general pactice. *Br. Med. J.*, **2**, 1115–1116

Devenyi, P. and Wilson, M. (1971). Abuse of barbiturates in an alcoholic population. *Can. Med. Assoc. J.*, **104**, 219–221.

Dobbie, J. A. (1982). Oxazepam withdrawal syndrome. *Med. J. Aust.*, **1**, 545

Downing, R. W. and Rickels, K. (1981). Coffee consumption, cigarette smoking and reporting of drowsiness in anxious patients treated with benzodiazepines or placebo. *Acta Psychiatr. Scand.*, **64**, 398–408

139

Durrant, B. W. (1965). Amphetamine addiction. *Practitioner*, **194**, 649–651

Dysken, M. W. and Chan, C. H. (1977). Diazepam withdrawal psychosis: a case report. *Am. J. Psychiatry*, **134**, 573

Ebihara, H. and Ikeda, R. (1978). A case who has taken chlordiazepoxide in a large quantity for a long time. *Clin. Psychiatry*, **20**, 1264–1266

Eddy, N. B., Halbach, H., Isbell, H. and Seevers, M. H. (1965). Drug dependence: its significance and characteristics. *Bull. WHO*, **37**, 1–12

Editorial (1975). Mental health in developing countries. *Br. Med. J.*, **4**, 187–188

Editorial (1984). Psychotherapy: effective treatment or expensive placebo. *Lancet*, **1**, 83–84

Edwards, J. G. and Glen-Bott, M. (1984). Does viloxazine have epileptogenic properties? *J. Neurol. Neurosurg. Psychiatry*, **47**, 960–964

Eichner, H. L. and Aebi, E. (1970). Septic retinitis due to injection of a homemade alcoholic beverage. *J. Am. Med. Assoc.*, **213**, 1644–1646

Einarson, T. R. (1980). Lorazepam withdrawal seizures. *Lancet*, **1**, 151

Endo, S., Kubota, I. and Kato, H. (1979). Withdrawal syndrome of nitrazepam in an elderly case. *Clin. Psychiatry*, **21**, 1117–1119

Epstein, R. S. (1980). Withdrawal symptoms from chronic use of low-dose barbiturates. *Am. J. Psychiatry*, **137**, 107–108

Essig, C. F., Jones, B. E. and Lam, R. C. (1969). The effect of pentobarbital on alcohol withdrawal in dogs. *Arch. Neurol.*, **20**, 554–558

Ewing, J. A. and Bakewell, W. E. (1967). Diagnosis and management of depressive drug dependence. *Am. J. Psychiatry*, **123**, 909–917

Fabre, L. F. and McLendon, D. M. (1980). Long term (6 month) safety and efficacy study of the benzodiazepines ketazolam and diazepam. *Clin. Res.*, **28**, 588A

Fabre, L. F., McLendon, D. M. and Harris, R. T. (1976). Preference studies of triazolam with standard hypnotics in out-patients with insomnia. *J. Int. Med. Res.*, **4**, 247–254

Facey, F. L., Weil, M. H. and Rosoff, L. (1966). Mechanism and treatment of shock associated with acute pancreatitis. *Am. J. Surg.*, **111**, 374–381

Feely, M., Calvert, R. and Gibson, J. (1982). Clobazam in catamenial epilepsy. *Lancet*, **2**, 71–73

Feuerlein, W. and Busch, H. (1972). Valiumsucht. *Internistische Praxis*, **12**, 349, 353

Finkle, B. S. McCloskey, K. L. and Goodman, L. S. (1979). Diazepam and drug associated deaths: a United States and Canadian survey. *J. Am. Med. Assoc.*, **242**, 429–434

Fleming, J. A. E. (1984). Triazolam abuse. *Can. Med. Assoc. J.*, **129**, 324–325

Floyd, J. B. Jr. and Murphy, C. M. (1976). Hallucinations following withdrawal of valium. *J. Kentucky Med. Assoc.*, **74**, 549–550

Fontaine, R., Chouinard, G. and Annable, L. (1984). Rebound anxiety in anxious patients after abrupt withdrawal of benzodiazepine treatment. *Am. J. Psychiatry*, **141**, 848–852

Fox, R. (1978). Abuse of benzodiazepines. *Lancet*, **2**, 681–682

Fraser, H. F., Essig, C. F. and Wolbach, A. B. Jr. (1961). Evaluation of carisoprodol and phenyramidol for addictiveness. *Bull. Narcotics*, **13**, 1

Fraser, H. F. and Jasinski, D. R. (1977). The assessment of the abuse potentiality of sedative/hypnotics (depressants) (methods used in the animals and man), In Martin, W. R. (ed.) *Handbook of Experimental Pharmacology*. Vol. 45, p. 589. (New York: Springer-Verlag)

Fraser, H. F. Wikler, A., Isbell, H. and Johnson, N. K. (1957). Partial equivalence of chronic alcohol and barbiturate intoxications. *Q. J. Stud. Alcohol.*, **18**, 541–551

Freed, A. (1976). Prescribing of tranquillisers and barbiturates by general practitioners. *Br. Med. J.*, **2**, 1232–1233

REFERENCES

Friedman, G. D., Siegelaub, A. B. and Seltzer, C. C. (1974). Cigarettes, alcohol, coffee and peptic ulcer. *N. Engl. J. Med.*, **290**, 469–473

Fruensgaard, K. (1976). Withdrawal psychosis: a study of 30 consecutive cases. *Acta Psychiatr. Scand.*, **53**, 105–118

Fruensgaard, K. and Vaag, U. H. (1975). Abstinenspsykose efter nitrazepam. *Ugesk. Laeger*, **137**, 633–634

Funderburke, F., McLeod, D., Griffiths, R. R. *et al.* (1983). Diazepam (DZ) and lorazepam (LZ): comparison of behavioral and subjective effects. *Pharmacologist*, **25**, 199

Gabriel, E. (1966). Valium in der nervenaerztlichen Praxis. *Wien Med. Wochenschr.*, **116**, 877–879

Gilbert, R. M. (1976). Caffeine as a drug of abuse. In Gibbin, R. G., Israel, Y. *et al.* (eds.). *Research Advances in Alcohol and Drug Problems.* (New York: John Wiley and Sons)

Gillberg, C. (1977). Diazepam intoxikation i nyfoddhetsperioden. *Laekertidningen*, **74**, 2587–2588

Gillie, O. (1975). *Sunday Times*, 7th December

Glatt, M. M. (1974). *A Guide to Addiction and its Treatment.* (Lancaster: MTP Press)

Glatt, M. M. and Marks, J. (eds.) (1982) *The Dependence Phenomenon.* (Lancaster: MTP Press)

Goldstein, A. (1972). Communication on the drug abuse problem. In Kunz, R. M. and Fehr, H. (ed.) *The Challenge of Life.* 335–344, and 96 (Basel: Birkhaeuser Verlag)

Golombok, S. and Lader, M. (1984). The psychopharmacological effects of premazepam, diazepam and placebo in healthy human subjects. *Br. J. Clin. Pharmacol.*, **18**, 127–133

Good, W. V. and Dubovsky, S. L. (1982). Pseudodementia masking substance abuse and depression. *Psychosomatics*, **23**, 656–657

Gordon, E. B. (1967). Addiction to diazepam (Valium). *Br. Med. J.*, **1**, 112.

Gossop, M. and Roy, A. (1977). Hostility, crime and drug dependence. *Br. J. Psychiatry*, **130**, 272–278

Gotestam, K. G. (1973). Intragastric self-administration of medazepam in rats. *Psychopharmacology*, **28**, 87

Grant, I. N. (1969). Drug habituation in an urban general practice. *Practitioner*, **202**, 428–430

Gray, J. A., Holt, L. and McNaughton, N. (1983). Clinical implications of the experimental pharmacology to the benzodiazepines. In Costa, E. (ed.) *The Benzodiazepines from Molecular Biology to Clinical Practice*, 147–172. (New York: Raven Press)

Greden, J. F. (1974). Anxiety or caffeinism: a diagnostic dilemma. *Am. J. Psychiatry*, **131**, 1089–1094

Greden, J. F., Procter, A. and Victor, B. (1981). Caffeinism associated with greater use of other psychotropic agents. *Comprehens. Psychiatry*, **22**, 565–571

Greenblatt, D. J., Allen, M. D., Noel, B. J. and Shader, R. I. (1977). Acute overdosage with benzodiazepine derivatives. *Clin. Pharm. Ther.*, **21**, 497–514

Greenblatt, D. J. and Shader, R. I. (1974). *Benzodiazepines in Clinical Practice.* (New York: Raven Press)

Greenblatt, D. J. and Shader, R. K. (1981). Clinical use of the benzodiazepines. *Rational Drug Therapy*, **15**, 1–6

Griffiths, R. R. and Ator, N. A. (1981). Benzodiazepine self-administration in animals and humans: a comprehensive literature review. In Szara, S. I. and Ludford, J. P. (eds.) *Benzodiazepines: a Review of Research Results.* NIDA Research Monograph No. 33, 37–61

Griffiths, R. R. and Bigelow, G. E. (1981). Human self-administration of sedative and stimulant drugs. *Psychopharmacol. Bull.*, **17**, 138–140

Griffiths, R. R., Bigelow, G. E. and Liebson, I. (1976). Human sedative self-administration: Effects of interingestion interval and dose. *J. Pharmacol. Exp. Ther.*, **197,** 488

Griffiths, R. R., Bigelow, C. E. and Liebson, I. (1979). Human drug self-administration, double-blind comparison of pentobarbital, diazepam, chlorpromazine and placebo. *J. Pharmacol. Exp. Ther.*, **210,** 301–310

Griffiths, R. R., Bigelow, G. E. and Liebson, I. (1983). Differential effects of diazepam and pentobarbital on mood and behaviour. *Arch. Gen. Psychiatry*, **40,** 865–873

Griffiths, R. R., Bigelow, G. E, Liebson, I. and Kaliszak, J. E. (1980). Drug preference in humans: double-blind choice comparison of pentobarbital, diazepam and placebo. *J. Pharmacol. Exp. Ther.*, **215,** 649–661

Griffiths, R. R., Lucas, S., Bradford, L. D. and Brady, J. V. (1981). Self-injection of barbiturates and benzodiazepines in baboons. *Psychopharmacology*, **75,** 101–109

Griffiths, R. R., McLeod, D. R. Bigelow, G. E. *et al.* (1984). Comparison of diazepam and oxazepam: Preference, liking and extent of abuse. *J. Pharmacol. Exp. Ther.*, **229,** 501–508

Grigor, J. M. G. (1982). Oxazepam withdrawal syndrome. *Med. J. Australia*, **1,** 288

Guile, L. A. (1963). Rapid habituation to chlordiazepoxide ('Librium'). *Med. J. Australia*, **50,** 56–57

Gunne, L. M. (1965). Om tillvaenjningsrisken vid medikamentell behandling av alkoholabstingens. *Nord. Psykiat. Tidskr.*, **19,** 352–357

Hackett, D. and Hall, J. M. (1977). Reinforcing properties of intravenous diazepam in rhesus monkeys (*Macaca mulatta*) with a history of codeine self-administration. *Proc. Europ. Soc. Toxicol.*, **18,** 308

Haefely, W. E., Kulcsar, A., Mohler, H., Pieri, L., Polc, P. and Schaffner, R. (1975). Possible involvement of GABA in the central actions of benzodiazepines. In Costa, E. and Greengard P. (eds.) *Mechanism of Action of Benzodiazepines.* pp. 131–151. (New York: Raven Press)

Haefely, W., Polc, P., Pieri, L. Schaffner, R. and Laurent, J.-P. (1983). Neuropharmacology of benzodiazepines: synaptic mechanisms and neural basis of action. In Costa, E. (ed.) *The Benzodiazepines: From Molecular Biology to Clinical Practice.* 21–66. (New York: Raven Press)

Hallberg, R. J. Lessler, K. Kane, F. J. (1964). Korsakoff-like Psychosis Associated with Benzodiazepine Overdosage. *Am. J. Psychiatry*, **121,** 188–189

Hallstrom, C. and Lader, M. (1981). Benzodiazepine withdrawal phenomena. *Int. Pharmacopsychiatry*, **16,** 235–244

Hanna, S. M. (1972). A case of oxazepam (Serenid D) dependence. *Br. J. Psychiatry*, **120,** 443–445

Harding, J. W. and Chrusciel, T. L. (1975). The use of psychotropic drugs in developing countries. *Bull. WHO*, **52,** 359–367

Harding, J. W., De Arango, M. V., Baltazar, J. *et al.* (1980). Mental disorders in primary health care: A study of their frequency and diagnosis in four developing countries. *Psychol. Med.*, **10,** 231–241

Harris, R. T., Claghorn, J. L. and Schoolar, J. C. (1968). Self-administration of minor tranquilizers as a function of conditioning. *Psychopharmacologia*, **13,** 81–90

Harrison, I. (1984). Drug addiction: the pharmacist's role. *Br. J. Pharmaceut. Pract.*, **6,** 372

Harrison, M., Busto, U., Naranjo, C. A. *et al.* (1984). Diazepam tapering in detoxification for high-dose benzodiazepine abuse. *Clin. Pharm. Ther.*, **36,** 527–533

Hartviksen, I. (1981). Er diazepinene sa uskyldige og forskrivningen 'blant norske leger sa moderat some ekspertisen gir uttrykk for? *Tidsskr. Nor. Laegenforen*, **101,** 595

Hasday, J. D. and Karch, F. E. (1981). Benzodiazepine prescribing in a family medical center. *J. Am. Med. Assoc.*, **246,** 1321–1325

REFERENCES

Haslerud, J. and Heskestad, S. (1981). Abstinens og forvirringsreaksjoner etter Rohypnol-bruk. *Tidsskr. Nor. Laegeforen*, **101**, 112

Hayashi, Y., Higashi, R. and Kadota, K. (1974). Three cases of chronic chlordiazepoxide intoxication with their withdrawal symptoms. *Clin. Psychiatry*, **16**, 77–82

Hayner, G. and Inaba, D. (1983). A pharmacological approach to outpatient benzodiazepine intoxication. *J. Psychoactive Drugs*, **15**, 99–104

Healey, M. L. and Pickens, R. W. (1983). Diazepam dose preference in humans. *Pharmacol. Biochem. Behav.*, **18**, 449–456

Hesbacher, P. Stepansky, P. Stepansky, E. and Rickels, K. (1976). Psychotropic drug use in family practice. *Pharmakopsychiat. Neuropsychopharmakol.*, **9**, 50–60

Hippius, H. E. and Ruther, F. (1982). Benzodiazepine, Mittel edr ersten Wahl. *Munch. Med. Wochenschr.*, **124**, 16–18

Hoff, H. and Hofmann, G. (1965). *Internat. Kong. der Internat. Soc. Hyg. Praeventivmedizin.*, Vienna, p. 35

Hoffmeister, F. (1977). Assessment of the reinforcing properties of stimulant and depressant drugs in the rhesus monkey as a tool for the prediction of dependence-producing capability in man. In Thompson, T. and Unna, K. (eds.). *Predicting Dependence Liability of Stimulant and Depressant Drugs.* p. 185. (Baltimore: University Park Press)

Hollister, L. E. (1975). Drugs for emotional disorders, current problems. *J. Am. Med. Assoc.*, **234**, 942–947

Hollister, L. E. (ed.). (1977). Valium. A discussion of current issues. *Psychosomatics*, **18**, 44–58

Hollister, L. E. (1980). Dependence on benzodiazepines. In Szara, S. I. and Ludford, J. P. (eds.). *Benzodiazepines: a review of research results.* NIDA Research Monograph, 33 Rockville, Maryland, pp. 70–82

Hollister, L. (1983). Principles of therapeutic application of the benzodiazepines. *J. Psychoactive Drugs*, **15**, 41–44

Hollister, L. E., Conley, F. K., Britt, R. H. and Schuer, L. (1980). Long-term use of diazepam, *J. Am. Med. Assoc.*, **246**, 1568–1570

Hollister, L. E., Motzenbecker, F. P. and Degan, R. O. (1961). Withdrawal reactions from chlordiazepoxide (Librium). *Psychopharmacologia*, **2**, 63–68

Holmberg, G. (1969). Misbrukas diazepam. Behandlung av oro, angest och soemnsvarigheter. *Laekartidningen*, **66**, 77–81

Holt, R. J. and Perez-Cruet, J. (1982). Hypersomnic diazepam abstinence syndrome: a case report. *Bol. Assoc. Med. Pr.*, **74**, 262–264

Hoover, J. P. (1972). College drug scene as it is. *New York State J. Med.*, **72**, 1886–1892

Hopkins, D. R., Sethi, K. B. S. and Mucklow, J. C. (1982). Benzodiazepine withdrawal in general practice. *J. R. Coll. Gen. Pract.*, **32**, 758–762

Howe, J. G. (1980). Lorazepam withdrawal seizures. *Br. Med. J.*, **1**, 1163–1164

Huxley, A. (1959). *The Doors of Perception and Heaven and Hell.* p. 51 (Harmondsworth: Penguin Books)

Idanpaan-Heikkila, J. (1979). *Studies in Drug Utilisation.* WHO Regional Publications European Series No. 8, Copenhagen, WHO

Illich, I. D. (1975). *Medical Nemesis.* (London: Calder & Boyars)

Illich, I. D. (1976). *Limits to Medicine: Medical Nemesis.* (London: Calder & Boyers)

Imoto, R. M. (1980). Benzodiazepine withdrawal reaction. *Drug Intell. Clin. Pharm.*, **14**, 187

Iswariah, V. (1966). Survey of the Problem of Habitual Drug Usage amongst the Public. *Trans. All-India Inst. Mental Hlth.*, **6**, 1–27

Jacquet, Y. F. and Stokes, D. (1975). Schedule-induced drug ingestion: differences due to type of drug. Paper presented at the annual meeting of the Eastern Psychological Association, New York

Jaffe, J. H., Ciraulo, D. A., Nies, A. *et al.* (1983). Abuse potential of halazepam and of diazepam in patients recently treated for acute alcohol withdrawal. *Clin. Pharmacol. Ther.*, **34**, 623–630

Jasinski, D. R. (1977). Assessment of the abuse potentiality of morphine-like drugs (methods used in man). In Martin, W. R. (ed.). *Handbook of Experimental Pharmacology.* Vol. 45, p. 197. (New York: Springer-Verlag)

Jasinski, D. R. and Johnson, A. E. (1982a) Abuse potential of diazepam (Valium). Abstract, Annual Meeting of American Society for Clinical Pharmacology and Therapeutics, Lake Buena Vista, Florida, 17 March

Jasinksi, D. R. and Johnson, R. E. (1982b). Abuse potential of chlordiazepoxide. *Pharmacologist*, **24**, 133

Jenkins, R. (1985). Women and minor psychiatric morbidity. *J. R. Soc. Med.*, **78**, 95–97

Jensen, H. H. and Poulsen, J. C. (1982). Amnesic effects of diazepam: drug dependence explained by state-dependent learning. *Scand. J. Psychol.*, **23**, 107–111

Jepsen, P. W. and Haastrup, S. (1979). Abstinensreaktioner efter benzodiazepiner. *Ugeskr. Laeg.*, **141**, 1121–1125

Jick, H., Slone, D., Dinan, B. and Muench, H. (1966). Evaluation of drug efficacy by a preference technique. *N. Engl. J. Med.*, **275**, 1399

Johanson, C. E. and Uhlenhuth, E. H. (1980). Drug preference and mood in humans: Diazepam. *Psychol. Pharmacol.*, **71**, 269

Johanson, C. E. and Uhlenhuth, E. H. (1982). Drug preferences in humans. *Fed. Proc.*, **41**, 228–233

Johnson, L. C. (1969). Psychological and physiological changes following total sleep deprivation. In Kales, A. A. (ed.). *Sleep – Physiology and Pathology.* pp. 206–220. (Philadelphia: Lippincott)

Jones, L., Simpson, D., Brown, A. C. *et al.* (1984). Prescribing psychotropic drugs in general practice: three year study. *Br. Med. J.*, **289**, 1045–1048

Kahan, B. B. and Haskett, R. F. (1984). Lorazepam withdrawal and seizures. *Am. J. Psychiatrt*, **141**, 1011–1012

Kaim, S. C. (1973). Benzodiazepines in the treatment of alcohol withdrawal states. In Garattini, S., Mussini, E. and Randall, L. O. (eds.) *The Benzodiazepines.* p. 571. (New York: Raven Press)

Kaim, S., Klett, C. J. and Rothfield, B. (1969). Treatment of the acute alcohol withdrawal state – a comparison of four drugs. *Am. J. Psychiatry*, **125**, 1640

Kales, A. Scharf, M. B., Kales, J. D. and Soldatos, C. R. (1979). Rebound insomnia: a potential hazard following withdrawal of certain benzodiazepines. *J. Am. Med. Assoc.*, **241**, 1692–1695

Kamano, D. K. and Arp, D. J. (1965). Chlordiazepoxide (Librium) consumption under stress conditions in rats. *Int. J. Neuropsychiatry*, **1**, 189

Kandel, D. B. and Logan, J. A. (1984). Patterns of drug use from adolescence to young adulthood. i. Periods of risk for initiation, continued use, and discontinuation. *Am. J. Publ. Health*, **74**, 660–666

Kaneto, H., Tsuchie, F. and Miyagawa, H. (1973). Attempt to evaluate the physical dependence liability of psychotropic drugs in mice. *Jpn. J. Pharmacol.*, **23**, 95P.

Kato, M. Takahashi, N., Miyagawa, K. *et al.* (1966). Clinical and statistical study on drug dependence, in particular induced by tranquillising and hypnotic drugs. *Clin. Psychiatry*, **2**, 1–12

Kawai, H. (1974). Drug toxicity in view of organ disturbance XVI. Central nervous system VI. *Pharm. Monthly*, **16**, 1488–1492

Kelleher, R. T. (1976). Characteristics of behaviour controlled by scheduled injections of drugs. *Pharmacol. Rev.*, **27**, 307

Kellermann, B. (1975). Uber Medikamenten-Abusus aus klinisch-psychiatrischer Sicht. *Hamburger Aerztebl.*, **29**, 28–29

REFERENCES

Kellett, J. M. (1974). The benzodiazepine bonanza. *Lancet*, **2**, 964

Kemper, N., Poser, W. and Poser, S. (1980). Benzodiazepin-Abhangigkeit. *Dtsch. Med. Wochenschr.*, **105**, 1707–1712

Keup, W. (1968). Abuse-liability and narcotic antagonism of pentazocine (report of two cases). *Dis. Nerv. Syst.*, **29**, 599–602

Keup, W. (1982). Pleasure seeking and the aetiology of drug dependence. In Glatt, M. M. and Marks, J. (eds.) *The Dependence Phenomenon*. pp. 1–20. (Lancaster: MTP Press)

Khan, A., Joyce, P. and Jones, A. V. (1980). Benzodiazepine withdrawal symptoms. *N.Z. Med. J.*, **92**, 94–96

Kielholz, P. (1968). Gesamtschweizerische Enquete ueber die Haeufigkeit des Medikamenten-Missbrauches. *Schweiz. Aerzte-Ztg.*, **49**, 1077–1096

Kielholz, P. (1971). Definition und Aetiologe der Drogenabhanackeit. *Bull. Schweiz. Akad. Wiss.*, **27**, 7–14

Kornblith, A. B. (1981). Multiple drug abuse involving nonopiate, nonalcoholic substances. 1. Prevalence. *Int. J. Addict.*, **16**, 197–232

Kornblith, A. B. and Shollar, E. (1978). The effect of chronic medical conditions in methadone maintenance patients on the course of their rehabilitation. In Smith, D. E. (ed.) *A Multicultural View of Drug Abuse*. (Proceedings of the National Drug Abuse Conf.). pp. 180–193. (Cambridge, Mass.: Schenkman)

Korsgaard, S. (1976). Misbrug af lorazepam (Temesta). *Ugeskr. Laeg.*, **138**, 164–165

Koumjian, K. (1981). The use of Valium as a form of social control. *Soc. Sci. Med.*, **15E**, 245–249

Koutsky, C. D. and Larson, T. G. (1967). Addiction cases treated on a psychiatric service. *Anesth. Analg. Curr. Res.*, **46**, 521–526

Kramer, J. C. (1978). Social benefits and social costs of drug control laws. *J. Drug Issues*, **8**, 1–7

Kryspin-Exner, K. (1966). Missbrauch von Benzodiazepinderivaten bei Alkoholkranken. *Br. J. Addict.*, **61**, 283–290

Kryspin-Exner, K. (1970). Alkoholismus und Medikamentenmissbrauch im Alter. In Doberauer, W. (ed.) *Geriatricum* pp. 305–314

Kryspin-Exner, K. and Demel, I. (1975). The use of tranquillizers in the treatment of mixed drug abuse. *Int. J. Clin. Pharmacol.*, **12**, 13

Krzyzowski, J. and Michniewicz, M. (1966). Przypadek Libriomania. *Neurol. Neurochir. Psychiat. Polska*, **16**, 195–196

Lader, M. H. (1969). *Studies of Anxiety*. (Ashford, Kent: Headley Bros.)

Lader, M. H. (1980a). New perspectives in benzodiazepine therapy: introduction. *Arzneim.-Forsch.*, **30**, 851

Lader, M. H. (1980b). The present status of benzodiazepines in psychiatry and medicine. *Arzneim.-Forsch.*, **30**, 910–912

Lader, M. (1982). Psychological effects of buspirone. *J. Clin. Psychiatry*, **43**, 62–67

Lader, M. H., Curry, S. and Baker, W. J. (1980). Physiological and psychological effects of clorazepate in man. *Br. J. Clin. Pharmacol.*, **9**, 83–90

Lader, M. and Petursson, H. (1983a). Rational use of anxiolytic/sedative drugs. *Drugs*, **25**, 514–528

Lader, M. and Petursson, H. (1983b). Long-term effects of benzodiazepines. *Neuropharmacology*, **22**, 527–533

Lader, M. H., Ron, M. and Petursson, H. (1984). Computed axial brain tomography in long-term benzodiazepine users. *Psycholog. Med.*, **14**, 203–206

Ladewig, D. (1973). Enquete sur l'ensemble du territoire Suisse concernant la frequence de l'abus des medicaments et des drogues. *Schweiz. Apotheker-Zeitung*, **111**, 548–551

Ladewig, D. Banzider, W. and Lownheck, M. (1981). Tranquillizer abuse – results of a nationwide Swiss survey. *TGO Tijdschrift voor Geneesmiddelenonderzoek.* **6,** 1132–1137

Lai, G. (1961). Toxicité du librium: observations après tentatives de suicide. *Med. Hyg.,* **19,** 685

Lande, A. (1970). Principles of effective drug abuse control. Paper presented at the International Institute on the Prevention and Treatment of Drug Dependence, pp. 51–79

Lapierre, Y. D. (1981). Benzodiazepine withdrawal. *Can. J. Psychiatry,* **26,** 93–95

Laporte, J. R., Capella, D., Gisbert, R., Porta, M. *et al.* (1981). The utilization of sedative-hypnotic drugs in Spain. In Tognoni, G. *et al.* (eds.) *Epidemiological Impact of Psychotropic Drugs.* (Amsterdam: Elsevier/North-Holland Biomedical Press)

Laughren, T. P., Battey, Y. W. and Greenblatt, D. J. (1982). Chronic diazepam treatment in psychiatric outpatients. *J. Clin. Psychiatry,* **43,** 461–462

Laux, G. (1979). Ewin Fall von Lexotanil – Athoengigkeit. Kasuistischer Beitrag zum Tranquilizermissbrauch. *Nervenarzt,* **50,** 326–327

Lawson, A. A. H. and Mitchell, I. (1972). Patients with acute poisoning seen in a general medical unit (1960-1971). *Br. Med. J.,* **4,** 153–156

Le Bellec, M., Bismuth, Ch., Lagier, G. and Dally, S. (1980). Syndrome de sevrage severe apres arret des benzodiazepines. *Therapie,* **35,** 113

Ledda, F. (1968). Intossicazzione acute da clordiazepossido in tossicomane seguita da sindrome astinenziale. *Clin. Ther.,* **44,** 167–171

Le Fevre, C. G. (1971). Drug dependence and drug abuse in New South Wales. *Med. J. Australia,* **58,** 715–716

Le Fevre, C. G. (1971). A factual study of drug dependence and drug abuse during 1965-1969 in New South Wales: a summary. *Med. J. Australia,* **58,** 395–397

Lennane, K. H. (1982a). Oxazepam withdrawal syndrome. *Med. J. Australia,* **1,** 545

Lennane, K. J. (1982b). Oxazepam withdrawal syndrome. *Med. J. Australia,* **1,** 287

Leung, F. W., Guze, P. A. (1983). Diazepam withdrawal. *West. J. Med.,* **138,** 98–101

Levy, A. B. (1984). Delirium and seizures due to abrupt alprazolam withdrawal: case report. *J. Clin. Psychiatry,* **45,** 38–39

Levy, R. M., Brown, A. R. and Halikas, J. A. (1972). Illicit pentazocine (Talwin) use: a report of thirteen cases. *Int. J. Addictions,* **7,** 693–700

Lingjaerde, O. (1964). Akute und Chronische Ueberdosierung von Diazepam (Valium). Paper presented at the Tagung der Norwegischen Psychiatrishcen Gesellschaft, Oslo/Nor. 23 October

Lingjaerde, O. (1965). Acute and chronic overdosage of diazepam (Valium). *Nord. Psykiat. Tidskr.,* **19,** 73–78

Lo, W. H. (1981). Personal communication.

Locket, S. (1973). Clinical toxicology. VII. Poisoning by salicylates, paracetamol, tricyclic anti-depressants and a miscellany of drugs. *Practitioner,* **211,** 105–112

Loveridge, P. L. (1981). Physical dependence on diazepam. *Can. Fam. Phys.,* **27,** 1109–1111

Lukas, S. E. and Griffiths, R. R. (1982a). Comparison of triazolam and diazepam self-administration by the baboon. *Pharmacologist,* **24,** 133

Lukas, S. E. and Griffiths, R. R. (1982b). Precipitated withdrawal in diazepam-treated baboons by a benzodiazepine receptor antagonist. *Fed. Proc.,* **41,** 1542

Lukas, S. E. and Griffiths, R. R. (1982c). Precipitated withdrawal by a benzodiazepine receptor antagonist (Ro 15-1788) after 7 days of diazepam. *Science,* **217,** 1161

Lukas, S. E. and Griffiths, R. R. (1984). Precipitated diazepam withdrawal in baboons: Effects of dose and duration of diazepam exposure. *Eur. J. Pharmacol.,* **100,** 163–171

Lunde, A. O. and Ropstad, O. (1970). Misbruk au lette ataratica. *Nord. Med.,* **85,** 655–658

REFERENCES

Lunde, P. K., Baksaas, I., Halse, M. *et al.* (1979). Studies in drug utilisation, WHO Regional Publications: European Series No. 8, Copenhagen, WHO

Lunde, P. K. M. (1977). Drug statistics and drug utilisation. In Colombo, J. *et al.* (eds.) *Epidemiological Evaluation of Drugs*. Proceedings of drugs symposium, Milan, 2-4 May,pp. 3-15. (Amsterdam: Elsevier/North Holland Biomedical Press)

Lupolover, R., Dazzi, H. and Ward, J. (1982). Rebound phenomena: results of a 10 years' (1970-1980) literature review. *Int. Pharmacopsychiatry*, **17**, 194–237

McCranie, E. W. (1978). Alleged sex-role stereotyping in the assessment of women's physical complaints: a study of general practitioners. *Soc. Sci. Med.*, **12**, 111–115

McNicholas, L. F. Martin, W. R. (1982a). Effects of Ro15-1788 (ethyl 8-fluoro-5, 6-dihydro-5-methyl-6-oxo-4H-imidazo [1, 5-A], [1, 4] benzodiazepine-3-carboxylate), a benzodiazepine antagonist, in diazepam (DZ)-dependent rats. *Fed. Proc.*, **41**, 1639

McNicholas, L. F. and Martin, W. R. (1982b). The effect of benzodiazepine antagonist, Ro15-1788 in diazepam dependent rats. *Life Sci.*, **31**, 731

McNicholas, L. F., Martin, W. R. and Cherian, S. (1982). Physical dependence on diazepam (D) and lorazepam (L) in the dog. *Pharmacologist*, **24**, 133

Mader, R. (1972). Primaere Valiumabhaengigkeit bei einem Jugendlichen. *Wiener Med. Wochenschr.*, **122**, 699–700

Malatinsky, J., Prochazka, M. and Kadlic, T. (1975). Transient psychological syndrome following diazepam therapy for tetanus. *Postgrad. Med. J.*, **51**, 860–863

Malcolm, M. T. (1972). Temporal lobe epilepsy due to drug withdrawal. *Br. J. Addict.*, **67**, 309–312.

Maletzky, B. M. (1974). Assisted covert sensitization for drug abuse. *Int. J. Addict.*, **9**, 411–429

Maletzky, B. M. and Klotter, J. (1976). Addiction to diazepam. *Int. J. Addict.*, **2**, 95–115

Manheimer, D. D., Davidson, S. T. and Balter, M. B. (1973). Popular attitudes and beliefs about tranquillizers. *Am. J. Psychiatry*, **130**, 1246–1253

Marjot, D. H. (1966). Drug dependence. *J. R. Nav. Med. Serv.*, **52**, 150–156

Marks, J. (1978). *The Benzodiazepines: Use, Overuse, Misuse, Abuse?* First Edn. (Lancaster: MTP Press)

Marks, J. (1980). The benzodiazepines – use and abuse. *Arzneim.-Forsch.*, **30**, 898–901

Marks, J. (1981). Diazepam – the question of long-term therapy and withdrawal reactions. *Drug Therapy*. Special Supplement.

Marks, J. (1982a). L'utilisation therapeutique des tranquillisants dans le monde. *Rev. Prat. (Paris)*, **32**, 2897–2908

Marks, J. (1982b). Benzodiazepine dependence in perspective. In Nicholson, A. N. (ed.) *Hypnotics in general practice*. pp. 67–73. (Oxford: Medicine Publishing Foundation)

Marks, J. (1982c). Dependence and psychoactive drugs. In Glatt, M. M. and Marks, J. (eds.) *The Dependence Phenomenon*. pp. 157–178. (Lancaster: MTP Press)

Marks, J. (1983a). The benzodiazepines – for good or evil. *Neuropsychobiology*, **10**, 115–126

Marks, J. (1983b). The benzodiazepines: an international perspective. *J. Psychoactive Drugs*, **15**, 137–149

Marks, J. (1983c). Measurement of the benefits of benzodiazepines. In Teeling Smith, G. (ed.) *Measuring the Social Benefits of Medicine*. pp. 128–138. (London: Office of Health Economics)

Marks, J. (1984). Stop it – I like it. *Rational Prescriber*, **4**, 1–3

Martin, P. R., Kapur, B. M, Whiteside, E. A. and Sellers, E. M. (1979). Intravenous phenobarbital therapy in barbiturate and other hypnosedative withdrawal reactions: a kinetic approach. *Clin. Pharmacol. Ther.*, **26**, 256–264

Martin, W. R. (ed.). (1977). *Drug Addiction. I. Handbook of Experimental Pharmacology*. p. 45. (New York: Springer-Verlag)

147

Martin, W. R. and McNicholas, L. F. (1981). *Benzodiazepine dependence studies in rodents, Benzodiazepines: A Review of Research Results, 1980.* (Research analysis and utilization system) Ed. by S. I. Szara and J. P. Ludford. *NIDA Research Monograph Series*, Vol. 33, p. 37

Martin, W. R., McNicholas, L. F. and Cherian, S. (1982). Diazepam and pentobarbital dependence in the rat. *Life Sci.*, **31**, 721

Maruta, T., Swanson, D. W. and Finlayson, R. E. (1979). Drug abuse and dependency in patients with chronic pain. *Mayo Clin. Proc.*, **54**, 241–244

Mayfield, D. G. and Montgomery, D. (1972). Alcoholism, alcohol intoxication, and suicide attempts. *Arch. Gen. Psychiatry*, **27**, 349–353

Mazzi, E. (1977). Possible neonatal diazepam withdrawal – a case report. *Am. J. Obstet. Gynecol.*, **129**, 586–587

Mellerio, F. (1980). Apport de l'electroencephalographie dans les accidents de sevrage des tranquillisants. *Rev. Electronceph. Neurophysiol. Clin.*, **10**, 95–103

Mellinger, G. D. (1978). Use of licit drugs and other coping alternatives: some personal observations on the hazards of living. In Lettiere, D.J. (ed.) *Drugs and Suicide – when other coping strategies fail.* (Beverly Hills: Sage Publications)

Mellinger, G. D. and Balter, M. B. (1981). Prevalence and patterns of use of psychotherapeutic drugs; results from a 1979 national survey of American adults. Paper, International Seminar on the Epidemiological Impact of Psychotropic Drugs, Milan, 24-26 June

Mellinger, G. D., Balter, M. B, Manheimer, D. I., Cisin, I. H. and Parry, H. J. (1978). Psychic distress, life crisis and the use of psychotherapeutic medications. *Arch. Gen. Psychiatry*, **35**, 1045–1052

Mellinger, G. D., Balter, M. B. and Uhlenhuth, E. H. (1984a). Prevalence and correlates of the long-term use of anxiolytics. *J. Am. Med. Assoc.*, **251**, 375–379

Mellinger, G. D., Balter, M. B. and Uhlenhuth, E. H. (1984b). Anti-anxiety agents: duration of use and characteristics of users in the USA. In: Rational Prescribing of Benzodiazepines. *Curr. Med. Res. Opin.* (Suppl. 4), **8**, 21–36

Mellor, L. S. and Jain, V. K. (1982). Diazepam withdrawal syndrome: its prolonged and changing nature. *Can. Med. Assoc. J.*, **127**, 1093–1096

Mendelson, G. (1978). Withdrawal symptoms after oxazepam. *Lancet*, **1**, 565

Merz, W. A. (1982). Standardized Assessment of the Symptoms of the Benzodiazepine Withdrawal Syndrome. 13th CINP Congress, Jerusalem, 20-25 June

Merz, W. A. and Ballmer, U. (1983). Symptoms of the barbiturate/benzodiazepine withdrawal syndrome in healthy volunteers: standardized assessment by a newly developed self-rating scale. *J. Psychoactive Drugs*, **15**, 71–84

Miller, F. and Nulsen, J. (1979). Diazepam (Valium) detoxification. *J. Nerv. Ment. Dis.*, **167**, 637–638

Miller, R. R. (1974). Hospital admissions due to adverse drug reactions – a report from the Boston Collaborative Drug Surveillance Program. *Arch. Int. Med.*, **134**, 219–223

Minter, R. and Murray, G. B. (1978). Diazepam withdrawal: a current problem in recognition. *J. Fam. Practice*, **7**, 1233–1235

Misra, P. C. (1975). Nitrazepam (Mogadon) dependence. *Br. J. Psychiatry*, **126**, 81–82

Miyasato, K. (1978). Experimental study on development of physical dependence on alcohol and cross physical dependence liability of diazepam and barbital to alcohol in rhesus monkeys. *Psychiat. Neurol. Jpn.*, **80**, 657

Moehler, H. and Okada, T. (1977). Benzodiazepine receptor: demonstration in the central nervous system. *Science*, **198**, 849–851

Moerck, H. J. and Magelund, G. (1979). Gynaecomastia and diazepam abuse. *Lancet*, **1**, 1344–1345

Moore, C. (1982). Oxazepam withdrawal syndrome. *Med. J. Australia*, **2**, 220

Morgan, B. B. (1974). Effects of continuous work and sleep loss in the reduction and recovery of work efficiency. *Am. Ind. Hyg. Assoc. J.*, **10**, 13–20

Morgan, H. G. (1984). Do minor affective disorders need medication?, *Br. Med. J.*, **289**, 783

Morgan, H. G., Bouluois, J. and Burns-Cox, C. (1973). Addiction to prednisone. *Br. Med. J.*, **2**, 93–94

Morgan, K. and Oswald, I. (1982). Anxiety caused by a short-life hypnotic. *Br. Med. J.*, **284**, 942

Morrison, A. A. (1974). Regulatory control of the Canadian Government over the manufacture, distribution and prescribing of psychotropic drugs. Cooperstock, R. (ed.) *Social aspects of the medical use of psychotropic drugs*. Addiction Research Foundation, Toronto, pp. 9–19

Morse, R. M. (1970). Postoperative deliria and emergency surgery: Dr. Morse replies. *Am. J. Psychiatry*, **126**, 1041

Muller, C. (1972). The overmedicated society: forces in the market place for medical care. *Science*, **76**, 489–492

Murphy, S. M., Owen, R. T. and Tyrer, P. J. (1984). Withdrawal symptoms after six weeks' treatment with diazepam. *Lancet*, **2**, 1389

Murray, J. (1981). Preliminary communication: long-term psychotropic drug-taking and the process of withdrawal. *Psycholog. Med.*, **11**, 853–858

Murray, J., Dunn, G., Williams, P. and Tarnopolsky, A. (1981). Factors affecting the consumption of psychotropic drugs. *Psychol. Med.*, **11**, 551–560

Nabarro, J. (1984). Unrecognised psychiatric illness in medical patients. *Br. Med. J.*, **289**, 635–636

Nagy, B. R. and Dillman, C. E. (1981). Case report of unusual diazepam abstinence syndrome. *Am. J. Psychiatry*, **138**, 694–695

Navaratnam, V. (1982). Impact of scheduling drugs under the 1971 convention on psychotropic substances – benzodiazepines reappraised, United Nations Research and Training Centre in Drug Dependence, National Drug Research Centre, Univ. Science Malaysia, Minden, Penang, Malaysia

Nerenz, K. (1974). Ein Fall von Valium-Entzugsdelir mit Grand-mal-Anfallen. *Nervenarzt*, **45**, 384–386

Newman, R. G. (1977). *Methadone Treatment in Narcotic Addiction: program management, findings and prospects for the future*. (New York: Academic Press)

Nicholson, A. N. and Marks, J. (1983). *Insomnia: A Guide for Practitioners*. (Lancaster: MTP Press)

Nicholson, A. N., Stone, B. M. and Spencer, M. B. (1982). Anxiety caused by a short-life hypnotic. *Br. Med. J.*, **284**, 1785

Nikolova, M., Daleva, L. and Nikolov, R. (1975). Study of tolerance to and barbiturate-like physical dependence on the tranquilizer Tempidon. *Agressologie*, **16**, 43

Noble, P. J. (1970). Drug-taking in delinquent boys. *Br. Med. J.*, **1**, 102–105

Norton, P. R. E. (1970). The effects of drugs on barbiturate withdrawal convulsions. *J. Pharm. Pharmacol.*, **22**, 763

Nurco, D. M. and Lerner, M. (1972). Drug abuse seen by physicians in a wealthy suburban county. In Report 34th Ann. Scient. Meet. Comm. problems of drug depend. Ann. Arbor, Mich., Natl. Acad. Sci., Natl. Res. Coun., pp. 643–658

O'Brien, J. (1978). The chemical trap – a patient's view. In: Dowsling, J. and Maclennan, A. (eds.) *The Chemical Dependent Woman, Rx, Recognition, Referral, Rehabilitation*. Proc. Conf. Dunwood Inst., Toronto Add. Res. Found., Toronto/Canada, pp. 49–55

Orrego, H., Blendis, L. M., Blake, J. E. *et al.* (1979). Reliability of assessment of alcohol intake based on personal interviews in a liver clinic. *Lancet*, **2**, 1354–1356

Oswald, I. (1982). Benzodiazepine hypnotics remain effective for 24 weeks. *Br. Med. J.*, **284**, 860–863

Oswald, I. and Priest, R. G. (1965). Five weeks to escape the sleeping pill habit. *Br. Med. J.*, **2**, 1093–1094

Parish, P. A., (1971). The prescribing of psychotropic drugs in general practice. *J. R. Coll. Gen. Pract.*, Suppl. 4, **21**

Parker, E. J. C. and Schreiber, V. (1980). Repeat prescribing – a study in one practice. *J. R. Coll. Gen. Pract.*, **30**, 603–606

Parry, H. J., Balter, M. B., Mellinger, G. D., Cisin, I. H. *et al.* (1973). National patterns of psychotherapeutic drug use. *Arch. Gen. Psychiatry*, **28**, 869–784

Parry, H. J., Cisin, I. H., Balter, M. B. *et al.* (1974). Increased alcohol intake as a coping mechanism for psychic distress. In Cooperstock, R. (ed.) *Social Aspects of the Medical Use of Psychotropic Drugs*. Addict. Res. Found., Toronto

Pearson, J., Baden, M. B. and Richter, R.W. (1974). Neuronal depletion in the Globus pallidus of heroin addicts. In 36th Annual Meeting Scientific Committee on Drug Dependence, Mexico City, pp. 187–199

Peck, A. W., Stern, W. C. and Watkinson, C. (1983). Incidence of seizures during treatment with tricyclic antidepressant drugs and bupropione. *J. Clin. Psychiatry*, **44**, 197–201

Peet, M. (1984). Beta-blockade in anxiety. *Postgrad. Med. J.*, **60**, 16–19

Perkins, M. E. and Bloch, H. I. (1970). Survey of a methadone maintenance program. *Am. J. Psychiatry*, **126**, 1389–1396

Peters, U. H. and Boeters, U. (1970). Valium-Sucht: eine Analyse anhand von 8 Faellen. *Pharmakopsychiat. Neuro-Psychopharmakol*, **3**, 339–348

Peters, U. H. and Seidel, M. (1970). Medikamentenmissbrauch und Sucht bei. *Arzneim. Forsch.*, **20**, 876–877

Petursson, H. and Lader, M. H. (1981a). Withdrawal from long-term benzodiazepine treatment. *Br. Med. J.*, **283**, 643–645

Petursson, H. and Lader, M. H. (1981b). Withdrawal reaction from clobazam. *Br. Med. J.*, **282**, 1932–1933

Petursson, H. and Lader, M. H. (1981c). Benzodiazepine dependence. *Br. J. Addict.*, **76**, 133–145

Petursson, H. and Lader, M. H. (1984). *Dependence on tranquillizers*. Maudsley Monograph No. 28. (Oxford: Oxford University Press)

Petzold, E. (1972). Valiumsucht. *Internist Praxis*, **12**, 355

Pevnick, J. S., Jasinski, D. R. and Haertzen, C. A. (1978). Abrupt withdrawal from therapeutically administered diazepam. *Arch. Gen. Psychiatry*, **35**, 995–998

Pichot, P. (1972). Disposibilité des drogues psychotropes et attitudes de la societé envers les troubles du comportment. In Kunz, R. M. and Fehr, H. (eds.) *The Challenge of Life*. pp. 85–89, 286–303. (Basel: Birkhauser Verlag)

Pickens, R. and Harris, W. C. (1968). Self-administration of d-amphetamine by rats. *Psychopharmacologia*, **12**, 158

Pihl, R. O., Marinier, R., Lapp, J. and Drake, H. (1982). Psychotropic drug use by women: characteristics of high consumers. *Int. J. Addict.*, **17**, 259–269

Poser, W., Poser, S., Roscher, D. and Argyrakis, A. (1983). Do benzodiazepines cause cerebral atrophy? *Lancet*, **1**, 715

Poshyachinda, V. (1982). Overview of diazepam abuse and implications for future social consequences. Institute of Health Research, Chulalongkorn Univ. Bangkok, Thailand. Tech. Rep. No. DD-3/82

Prescott, L. P. (1983). Safety of the benzodiazepines. In Costa, E. (ed.) *The Benzodiazepines: from molecular biology to clinical practice*. pp. 253–266. (New York: Raven Press)

Preskorn, S. H. and Denner, L. J. (1977). Benzodiazepines and withdrawal psychosis: Report of three cases. *J. Am. Med. Assoc.*, **237**, 36–38

REFERENCES

Preston, K. L., Griffiths, R. R., Stitzer, M. L. *et al.* (1984). Diazepam and methadone interactions in methadone maintenance. *Clin. Pharm. Ther.*, **36**, 534–541

Primm, B. (1981). Street preferences. FDA Drug Abuse Advis. Comm. Proc. of the meeting in Rockville, MD, 14-15 May, Vol. 2, pp. 98–104

Proctor, R. C. (1981). Prescription medication in the workplace. *North Carolina Med. J.*, **42**, 545–547

Quitkin, F. M., Rifkin, A., Kaplan, J. and Klein, D. F. (1972). Phobic anxiety syndrome complicated by drug dependence and addiction. *Arch. Gen. Psychiatry*, **27**, 159–162

Rane, A., Sundwall, A. and Tomson, G. (1979). Oxazepamabstinens i nyfoeddlets-perioden. *Laekartidningen*, **76**, 4416–4417

Raskind, M. and Bradford, T. (1975). Methylphenidate (Ritalin) abuse and methadone maintenance. *Dis. Nerv. Syst.*, **36**, 9–12

Rastogni, R. B., Lapierre, Y. D. and Singhal, R. L. (1978). Some neurochemical correlates of 'rebound' phenomenon observed during withdrawal after long-term exposure to 1,4-benzodiazepines. *Prog. Neuro-Psychopharmacol.*, **2**, 43–54

Ratna, L. (1981). Addiction to temazepam. *Br. Med. J.*, **282**, 1827–1828

Rechenberger, H. G. (1972). Valiumsucht. *Internistische Praxis*, **12**, 349, 354

Reeve, A. M. (1972). Treatment of persons addicted to or dependent on drugs. *J. Iowa Med. Soc.*, **62**, 436–437

Reigel, C. E. and Bourn, W. M. (1982). Low incidence of audiogenic convulsions upon withdrawal of diazepam cross-substituted for sodium barbital in dependent rats. *Fed. Proc.*, **41**, 1542

Relkin, R. (1966). Death following withdrawal of diazepam. *N.Y. State J. Med.*, 1770-1772

Rementeria, J. L. and Bhatt, K. (1977). Withdrawal symptoms in neonates from intrauterine exposure. *J. Pediat.*, **90**, 123–126

Remschmidt, H. and Dauner, I. (1970a). Klinische und Soziale Aspekte der Drogen-abhaengigkeit bei Jugendlichen. Teil 1. *Med. Klin.*, **65**, 1993–1997

Remschmidt, H. and Dauner, I. (1970b). Klinische und Soziale Aspekte der Drogen-abhaengigkeit bei Jugendlichen. Teil 2. *Med. Klin.*, **65**, 2041–2047

Rickels, K. (1981). Diazepam: the question of long-term therapy and withdrawal reactions. *Drug Therapy.* (Spec. Suppl.), 5–30

Rickels, K. (1982). Benzodiazepines in the treatment of anxiety. *Am. J. Psychother.*, **36**, 358–370

Rickels, K. (1983). Benzodiazepines in the treatment of anxiety: North American experience. In Costa, E. (ed.) *The Benzodiazepines: from Molecular Biology to Clinical Practice.* pp. 295–310. (New York: Raven Press)

Rickels, K. (1984). Paper presented at CINP Satellite meeting. 'Chronic treatments in neuro-psychiatry, Montecatini, 24-26 June

Rickels, K. and Brand, M. E. (1969). Incidence of non-narcotic drug addictions at a large city hospital. In Cole, J. O. and Wittenborn, J.R. (eds.) *Drug Abuse – Social and Psychopharmacological Aspects.* p. 49. (Springfield, Ill.: Charles C. Thomas)

Rickels, K., Case, W. G. and Diamond, L. (1980). Relapse after short-term drug therapy in neurotic outpatients. *Int. Pharmacopsychiatry*, **15**, 186–192

Rickels, K., Case, W. G. and Downing, R. W. (1982). Issues in long-term treatment with diazepam. *Psychopharmacol. Bull.*, **18**, 38–41

Rickels, K., Case, W. G., Downing, R. W. and Winokur, A. (1983). Long-term diazepam therapy and clinical outcome. *J. Am. Med. Assoc.*, **250**, 767–771

Rickels, K. *et al.* (1977). Halazepam and diazepam in neurotic anxiety: A double-blind study. *Psychopharmacology*, **52**, 129–136

Rifkin, A., Klein, D. F. and Quitkin, F. (1977). Withdrawal from diazepam. *J. Am. Med. Assoc.*, **238**, 306

151

Rifkin, A., Quitkin, F. and Klein, D. F. (1976). Withdrawal reaction to diazepam. *J. Am. Med. Assoc.*, **236**, 2172–2173

Roache, J. D. and Griffiths, R. R. (1983). Effects of diazepam (DZ), oxazepam (OX), triazolam (TZ), and phenobarbital (PB) on objective and subjective measures – assessment of abuse liability. *Pharmacologist*, **25**, 214

Roache, J. D. and Griffiths, R. R. (1984). Subjective and amnesic effects of triazolam (TZ) and pentobarbital (PB). *Fed. Proc.*, **43**, 931

Robinson, G. M. and Sellers, E. M. (1982). Diazepam withdrawal seizures. *Can. Med. Assoc. J.*, **126**, 944–945

Rosenberg, H. C. and Chiu, T. H. (1982). An antagonist-induced benzodiazepine abstinence syndrome. *Eur. J. Pharmacol.*, **81**, 153

Roskies, E. (1978). Sex, culture and illness – an overview. *Soc. Sci. Med.*, **12B**, 139–44

Rothstein, E., Cobble, J. C. and Sampson, N. (1976). Chlordiazepoxide: long-term use in alcoholism. *Ann. N.Y. Acad. Sci.*, **273**, 381–384

Royal College of Physicians (1983). *Health or Smoking*. Royal College of Physicians' Report. (London: Pitman)

Rümmele, W. (1968). Zeitliche Zusammenhaenge zwischen Erkrankungen, Operationen oder Unfaellen und dem Ausbruch eines Delirium Tremens. *Schweiz. Arch. Neurol. Neurochir. Psychiat.*, **101**, 192–200

Runge, M., Arnold, W. and Schreiber, D. (1971). Aktuelle Formen der drogenabhaengigkeit unter Besonderer Beruecksichtigung von Haschisch und LSD. *Med. Welt*, **22**, 1301–1308

Ryan, G. P. and Boisse, N. R. (1979). Production of benzodiazepine physical dependence in rats. *Pharmacologist*, **21**, 152

Saeny, E. C., Harvey, W. H., Oss, J. N., Turk, R. F. and Ginther, M. E. (1977). Adjunctive drug use by methadone patients. *Am. J. Drug Alcohol Abuse*, **4**, 533–541

Sereny, G. and Kalant, H. (1965). Comparative clinical evaluation of chlordiazepoxide and promazine in treatment of alcohol-withdrawal syndrome. *Br. Med. J.*, **1**, 92

Shinfuku, (1979). Long-term continued administration of sleep inducer – nitrazepam. *Jpn. Med. J.*, **136**

Säker, G. (1968). Ihr Fakll – und ihre Diagnose. *Aertz. Praxis*, **20**, 48

Salkind, M. R. (1981). Anxiety in the community. In Murray, R., Ghodse, H. *et al.* (eds.) *The Misuse of Psychotropic Drugs*. (Gaskell: R. Coll. Psychiatrists)

Sandman, A. R. (1976). Drug addiction. *Osteopath Annals*, **4**, 63, 65–68

Sanger, D. J. (1977). Schedule-induced drinking of chlordiazepoxide solutions by rats. *Pharmacol. Biochem. Behav.*, **7**, 1

Sardemann, H. and Friis-Hansen B. (1975). Nyfodte Bron af Narkomodre. *Ugesk. Laeger*, **137**, 859–863

Schopf, J. (1981). Long-term use of benzodiazepines: an unusual withdrawal syndrome may appear. Third World Cong. Biol. Psychiat., Stockholm

Schuster, C. B. and Thompson, T. (1969). Self administration of and behavioral dependence on drugs. *Ann. Rev. Pharmacol.*, **9**, 483

Schuster, C. L. and Humphries, R. H. (1981). Benzodiazepine dependency in alcoholics. *Connecticut med.*, **45**, 11–13

Selig, J. W. (1966). A possible oxazepam abstinence syndrome. *J. Am. Med. Assoc.*, **198**, 951–952

Sellers, E. M. and Busto, U. (1983). Diazepam withdrawal syndrome. *Can. Med. Assoc. J.*, **129**, 97

Sellers, E. M., Marsham, J. A., Kaplan, H. L. *et al.* (1981). Acute and chronic drug abuse emergencies in Metropolitan Toronto. *Int. J. Addict.*, **16**, 283–303

Sievewright, N. and Tyrer, P. J. (1984). Use of beta-blocking drugs in withdrawal states. *Postgrad. Med. J.*, **60**, 47–50

REFERENCES

Simon, P. (1983). Antidepressants, benzodiazepines, and convulsions. *Biol. Psychiatry*, **18,** 517

Sironi, V. A., Franzini, A., Ravagnati, L. and Marossero, F. (1979). Interictal acute psychoses in temporal lobe epilepsy during withdrawal of anticonvulsant therapy. *J. Neurol. Neurosurg. Psychiatry*, **42,** 724–730

Sironi, V. A., Miserocchi, G. and De Riu, P. L. (1984). Clonazepam withdrawal syndrome. *Acta Neurol (Napoli)*, **6,** 134–139

Sjoe, O., Hvidberg, E. F, Naestoft, J. and Lund, M. (1975). Pharmacokinetics and side-effects of clonazepam and its 7-amino metabolite in man. *Eur. J. Clin. Pharmacol.*, **8,** 249–254

Skinner, P. T. (1984). Skills not pills: learning to cope with anxiety symptoms. *J. R. Coll. Gen. Practit.*, **34,** 258

Slater, J. (1966). Suspected dependence on chlordiazepoxide hydrochloride (Librium). *Can. Med. Assoc. J.*, **95,** 416

Smith, A. J. (1972). Self poisoning with drugs: a worsening situation. *Br. Med. J.*, **4,** 157–159

Smith, D. E. (1979). Valium and low dose withdrawal syndrome. *J. Drug Alcohol Depend.*, **3,** 7–8

Smith, D. E. and Marks, J. (1985). Abuse of the benzodiazepines. In Smith, D. E. and Wesson, D. R. (eds.) *The Benzodiazepines*. (Lancaster: MTP Press)

Smith, D. E. and Wesson, D. R. (1983). Benzodiazepine dependency syndromes. *J. Psychoactive Drugs*, **15,** 85–96

Sokolow, L., Welte, J., Hynes, G. and Lyons, J. (1981). Multiple substance use by alcoholics. *Br. J. Addict.*, **76,** 147–158

Soueiff, M. I. (1981). The psychotropic convention in Egypt. In Smart, R. G, Murray, G. F. and Archibald, H. D. (eds.) *Psychotropic Substances and their International Control*. pp. 61–68. (Toronto: Alcoholism and Drug Addiction Research Foundation)

Spencer, P. S. J. (1981). Personal communication

Squires, R. and Braestrup, C. (1977). Benzodiazepine receptors in rat brain. *Nature*, **266,** 732–734

Stepney, R. (1980). *World Medicine*, 15 September

Stewart, R. B., Salem, R. B. and Springer, P. K. (1980). A case of lorazepam withdrawal. *Am. J. Psychiatry*, **137,** 1112–1114

Stitzer, M. L., Griffiths, R. R., McLellan, A. T. *et al.* (1981). Diazepam use among methadone maintenance patients: patterns and dosages. *Drug Alcohol Depend.*, **8,** 189–199

Stolerman, I. P., Kumar, R. and Steinberg, H. (1971). Development of morphine dependence in rats: lack of effect of previous ingestion of other drugs. *Psychopharmacologia*, **20,** 321

Sturmer, W. Q. and Garriott, J. C. (1973). Deaths involving propoxyphene. A study of 41 cases over a two-year period. *J. Am. Med. Assoc.*, **233,** 1125–1130

Sumiyoshi, S., Tsuzuki, J. (1977). A case presenting marked withdrawal symptoms after prolonged nitrazepam medication. *Kyorhu J. Psychiatry*, **23,** 234

Suzuki, T. Fukumori, R., Yoshii, T. *et al.* (1980). Effect of p-chlorophenylalanine on diazepam withdrawal signs in rats. *Psychopharmacology*, **71,** 91

Swain, H. (1983). Personal communication quoted in J. H. Woods. *Experimental abuse liability of benzodiazepines*. *J. Psychoactive Drugs*, **15,** 61–65

Swanson, D. W., Weddige, R. L. and Morse, R. M. (1973). Abuse of prescription drugs. *Mayo Clin. Proc.*, **48,** 359–367

Tagashira, E., Izumi, T. and Yanaura, S. (1977). Studies on drug dependence (report 24) methodological approach for drug dependence test of sedative-hypnotic drugs by daf-method. *Jpn. J. Pharmacol.*, **27,** 81P

Tagaya, M. and Koshino, Y. (1979). Withdrawal reaction to nitrazepam. *Jpn. Med. J.*, 43–47

Tait, I. and Hutchinson, E. C. (1977). An addiction to drug treatment. *Br. Med. J.*, **1**, 40–42

Takahashi, N., Miyagawa, K., Tauchi, K., Fujita, E. and Konda, Y. (1965). Dependence of chlordiazepoxide – with special reference to cases demonstating hallucinatory – delusional state after withdrawal. *Jpn. Med. J.*, **2163**, 31–34

Tallman, J. F., Paul, S. M. and Skolnick, P. (1980). Receptors for the age of anxiety: pharmacology of the benzodiazepines. *Science*, **207**, 274–276

Taylor, K. M. and Laverty, R. (1969). The effect of chlordiazepoxide, diazepam and nitrazepam on catecholamine metabolism in regions of the rat brain. *Eur. J. Pharmacol.*, **8**, 296–301

Teal, J. S. (1980). Comments on benzodiazepine reaction. *Drug. Intel. Clin. Pharm.*, **14**, 723

Teeling Smith, G. (ed.). (1983). *Measuring the Social Benefits of Medicine.* (London: Office of Health Economics)

Teigen, A. (1961). *Tidsk. Norsk. Laegeforen.*, **81**, 1375

Tennant, F. S. (1979). Outpatient treatment and outcome of prescription drug abuse. *Arch. Intern. Med.*, **139**, 154–156

Teo, S. H., Chee, K. T. and Tan, C. T. (1979). Psychiatric complications of Rohypnol abuse. *Singapore Med. J.*, **20**, 270

Tessler, J. F., Stokes, S. R. and Pietras, M. (1978). Consumer response to Valium. A survey of attitudes and patterns of use. *Drug. Ther.*, **8**, 179–186

Thompson, T. and Pickens, R. (1969). Drug self-administration and conditioning. In Steinberg, H. (ed.) *Scientific Basis of Drug Dependence.* p. 177. (London: Churchill)

Thompson, T. and Pickens, R. (1970). In Harris, R. T., McIsaac, W. M. and Schuster, C. R. (eds.). *Drug Dependence.* p. 143. (Austin: University of Texas Press)

Trickett, S. (1984). Personal communication.

Tsuchie, F., Nakanishi, H. and Kaneto, H. (1972). Attempt to evaluate the physical dependence liability of psychotropic drugs in mice. *Jpn. J. Pharmacol..* **22**, 92P

Twaddle, A. C. and Sweet, R. H. (1970). Characteristics and experiences of patients with preventable hospital admission. *Soc. Sci. Med.*, **4**, 141–145

Tyrer, P. (1974). The benzodiazepine bonanza. *Lancet*, **2**, 709

Tyrer, P. (1980). Lorazepam withdrawal seizures. *Lancet*, **1**, 151

Tyrer, P., Owen, R. and Dowling, S. (1983). Gradual withdrawal of diazepam after long-term therapy. *Lancet*, **1**, 1402-1406

Tyrer, P., Rutherford, D. and Huggett, T. (1981). Benzodiazepine withdrawal symptoms and propranolol. *Lancet*, **1**, 520–522

Tyrer, P., Steinberg, P. and Watson, B. (1980). Possible epileptogenic effect of mianserin. *Lancet*, **2**, 798–799

Tyrer, P. and Sievewright, N. (1984). Identification and management of benzodiazepine dependence. *Postgrad. Med. J.*, **60**, 41–46

Uhlenhuth, E. H. (1983). The benzodiazepines and psychotherapy: controlled studies of combined treatment. In Costa, E. (ed.) *The Benzodiazepines: from Molecular Biology to Clinical Practice.* pp. 325–338. (New York: Raven Press)

Uhlenhuth, E. H., Balter, M. B. and Lipman, R. S. (1978). Minor tranquilizers: clinical correlates of use in an urban population. *Arch. Gen. Psychiatry*, **35**, 650-655

Uhlenhuth, E. H., Balter, M. B., Mellinger, G. D. *et al.* (1984). Anxiety disorders: prevalence and treatment. In Rational prescribing of benzodiazepines. *Curr. Med. Res. Opin.* (Suppl. 4), **8**, 37–47

Uhlenhuth, E. H., Johanson, C. E., Kilgore, K. *et al.* (1981). Drug preference and mood in humans: preference for d-amphetamine and subject characteristics. *Psychopharmacology*, **74**, 191–194

REFERENCES

UNO (1971a). Convention of Psychotropic Substances, 1971. (New York: United National Organization)

UNO (1971b). United Nations: Commentary on the Convention on Psychotropic Substances. (New York: United Nations Organization)

UNO (1982). Report of the Seventh Special Session of the Commisssion on Narcotic Drugs. (Vienna: United Nations Organization)

UNO (1983). Report of the Thirtieth Session of the Commission on Narcotic Drugs. (Vienna: United Nations Organization)

UNO (1984). Report of the Eighth Special Session of the Commission on Narcotic Drugs. (Vienna: United Nations Organization)

Urban, H. (1964). Schoeden am Zentralnervensystem durch Missbrauch phenacetinhaltiger Mischpraeparate. *Dtsch. Med. Wochnschr.*, **89**, 223–229

Vaag, U. H. (1970). Lettere Abstinenssymptomer. *Ugeskr. Laeg.*, **132**, 1875–1877

Vaag, U. H. (1975). Abstinenspsykose i Tilslutning til Indsaettelse i Faengselsinstitution. *Ugeskr. Laeg.*, **137**, 634–635

Van Oefele, K., Wolf, B. and Ruther, T. (1983). Poster presentation at 4th International Cong. Sleep Res. Bologna, Italy, 18-22 July

Venzlaff, U. (1972). Ueber Valiummissbrauch und Valiumsucht. *Internist. Prax.*, **12**, 349–352

Verbrugge, L. M. (1978). Complaints and diagnoses: sex differences in the vocabulary and attribution of illness. Paper presented at the Amer. Publ. Health Assoc. Meet., Los Angeles

Vyas, I. and Carney, M. W. (1975). Diazepam withdrawal fits. *Br. Med. J.*, **1**, 44

Walters, L. and Nel, P. (1981) Die afhanklikheidspotensiaal van die benzodiasepiene. *S. Afr. Med. J.*, **59**, 115–116

Walton, N. U. and Deutsch, J. A. (1978). Self-administration of diazepam by the rat. *Behav. Biol.*, **24**, 533

Ward, J. (1980). *Social Aspects of Benzodiazepine Prescribing Today*. (Basel: Editiones Roche)

Wätzig, H. and Michaelis, R. (1973). Tavor: Kein problemloses Benzodiazepin-Derivat. *Nervenarzt*, **44**, 499–500

Weaver, S. S., Phillip, P. E. and Altshuler, H. L. (1975). Intragastric self-adminstration of sedative-hypnotic drugs by the rhesus monkey. *Pharmacologist*, **17**, 211

Weeks, J. R. (1962). Experimental morphine addiction: method for automatic intravenous injections in unrestrained rats. *Science*, **138**, 143–144

Weizel, A. (1973). Drogenmissbrauch aus der Sicht des Internisten. *Therapiewoche*, **22**, 3727–3733

Werner, R. E., Smith, S. G. and Davis, W. M. (1976). A dose–response comparison between methadone and morphine self-administration. *Psychopharmacology*, **47**, 209

WHO (1950). WHO definitions, WHO Expert Committee on Drugs liable to produce Addiction. Report on the 2nd Session. Tech. Rep. Ser. No. 21. (Geneva: WHO)

WHO (1964). WHO Definitions, WHO Expert Committee on Drugs liable to produce Addiction. Report on the 13th Session. Tech. Rep. Ser. No. 273. (Geneva: WHO)

WHO (1969). Expert Committee on Drug Dependence, 16th Report. World Health Org. Tech. Rep. Ser. No. 407. (Geneva: WHO)

WHO (1975). Evaluation of dependence liability and dependence potential of drugs: Report of a WHO Scientific Group. Tech. Res. Ser. No. 577. (Geneva: WHO)

WHO (1978). World Health Organisation Expert Committee on Drug Dependence, 21st Report. Tech. Rep. Ser. No. 618. (Geneva: WHO)

WHO (1981a). Report of the 5th World Health Organisation Review of Psychoactive Substances for International Control, 16th November. (Geneva: WHO)

WHO (1981b). Assessment of public health and social problems associated with the use of psychotropic drugs. Report of the WHO Expert Committee on Implementation of the Convention on Psychotropic Substances. Tech. Rep. Ser. No. 656. (Geneva: WHO)

WHO (1982). Report of the 6th World Health Organisation Review of Psychoactive Substances for International Control. (Geneva: WHO)

WHO (1983). Report of the 8th World Health Organisation Review of Psychoactive Substances for International Control, September. (Geneva: WHO)

Whybrow, P. C., Matlins, S. M. and Greenberg, M. D. (1982). The social impact of psychotropic drugs. Personal communication

Wilbur, R. and Kulik, A. V. (1983). Abstinence syndrome from therapeutic doses of oxazepam. Can. J. Psychiatry, 28, 298–300

Williams, P., Murray, J. and Clare, A. (1982). A longitudinal study of psychotropic drug prescription. Psychol. Med., 12, 201–206

Winokur, A. and Rickels, K. (1981). Withdrawal and pseudo-withdrawal from diazepam therapy. J. Clin. Psychiatry, 42, 442–444

Winokur, A. and Rickels, K. (1984). Withdrawal responses to abrupt discontinuation of desmethyldiazepam. Am. J. Psychiatry, 141, 1427–1429

Winokur, A. , Rickels, K., Greenberg, D. J. et al. (1980). Withdrawal reaction from long-term, low-dosage administration of diazepam. Arch. Gen. Psychiatry, 37, 101–105

Winstead, D. K., Anderson, A., Eilers, K. et al. (1974). Diazepam on demand: Drug seeking behavior in psychiatric inpatients. Arch. Gen. Psychiatry, 30, 349

Woimant, F., de Liege, Dorey, F. et al. (1983). Sevrage aux benzodiazepines. Complication par coma avec rigidite de decerebration. Presse Med., 12, 2765

Wolf, G., Jacquet, Y. and Carol, J. (1978). Test for oral and postingestional factors mediating differential acceptability of morphine, methamphetamine, and chlordiazepoxide drinking solutions. Psychopharmacology, 60, 101

Woods, J. H. (1983). Experimental abuse liability of benzodiazepines. J. Psychoactive Drugs, 15, 61–66

Woody, G. E., O'Brien, C. P. and Greenstein, R. (1975). Misuse and abuse of diazepam – an increasingly common medical problem. Int. J. Addict., 10, 843–848

Worm, K. and Schou, J. (1970). Narkomandodsfald. Ugesk. Laeger, 132, 1955–1960

Yamaguchi, K. and Kandel, D. B. (1984a). Patterns of drug use from adolescence to young adulthood. ii. Sequences of progression. Am J. Publ. Hlth., 74, 668–672

Yamaguchi, K. and Kandel, D. B. (1984b). Patterns of drug use from adolescence to young adulthood. iii. Predictions of progression. Am. J. Publ. Hlth., 74, 673–681

Yamasaki, M., Nomura, S. and Kimura, N. (1977). EEG on a case of diazepam abuse. Clin. Electroenceph., 19, 760–761

Yamashita, I. (1981). Paper read at the 4th S.E. Asia Psychotropics Meeting – Philippines

Yamashita, I. and Asano, Y. (1982). Survey of use of psychotropic agents in Asian Countries in 1978. Personal communication

Yanagita, T. (1973). An experimental framework for evaluation of dependence liability of various types of drugs in monkeys. Bull. Narcotics, 25, 57

Yanagita, T. (1981). Dependence-producing effects of anxiolytics. In Hoffmeister, F. and Stille, G. (eds.) Psychotropic Agents. Part II: Anxiolytics, Gerontopsychopharmacological Agents, and Psychomotor Stimulants. p. 395. (New York: Springer-Verlag)

Yanagita, T. (1983). Dependence potential of zopiclone studies in monkeys. Pharmacology, 27, 216–227

Yanagita, T. and Kato, S. (1982). Dependence studies on zopiclone. Paper presented at CPDD Meeting, Toronto, Canada

Yanagita, T., Kato, S. and Miyasato, K. (1981a). Dependence potential of flunitrazepam tested in rhesus monkeys. *CIEA* (Central Institute for Experimental Animals). *Preclinical Reports*, **7**, 37

Yanagita, T. and Kiyohara, H. (1976). Drug dependence potential of ID-540 tested in rhesus monkey. *CIEA Preclinical Reports*, **2**, 187

Yanagita, T., Miyasato, K. and Kiyohara, H. (1977a). Drug dependence potential of triazolam tested in rhesus monkeys. *CIEA Preclinical Reports*, **1**, 1

Yanagita, T., Miyasato, K. Takahashi, S. and Kiyohara, H. (1977b). Dependence potential of dipotassium clorazepate tested in rhesus monkeys. *CIEA Preclinical Reports*, **3**, 67

Yanagita, T. and Oinuma, N. (1982). Influence of physical dependence on reinforcing intensity of diazepam tested by the progressive ratio method in rhesus monkeys. ISGIDAR Meeting, Toronto, Canada, 27 June

Yanagita, T., Oinuma, N. and Nakanishi, H. (1981b). Drug dependence potential of clonazepam tested in the rhesus monkey. *CIEA Preclinical Reports*, **7**, 29

Yanagita, T., Oinuma, N. and Takahashi, S. (1975a). Drug dependence potential of Sch. 12041 (halazepam) evaluated in the rhesus monkey. *CIEA Preclinical Reports*, **1**, 231

Yanagita, T. and Takahashi, S. (1970). Development of tolerance to and physical dependence on barbiturates in rhesus monkeys. *J. Pharmacol. Exper. Ther.*, **172**, 163

Yanagita, T., and Takahashi, S. (1973). Dependence liability of several sedative-hypnotic agents evaluated in monkeys. *J. Pharmacol. Exp. Ther.*, **187**, 307

Yanagita, T., Takahashi, S., Ito, Y. and Miyasato, K. (1975b). Drug dependence potential of prazepam evaluated in the rhesus monkey. *CIEA Preclinical Reports*, **1**, 257

Yanagita, T., Takahashi, S., Nakanishi, H. and Oinuma, N. (1975e). Drug dependence potential of cloxazolazepam (cloxazolam) evaluated in the rhesus monkey. *CIEA Preclinical Reports*, **1**, 223

Yanagita, T., Takahashi, S., and Oinuma, N. (1975c). Drug dependence potential of lorazepam (WY 4036) evaulated in the rhesus monkey. *CIEA Preclinical Reports*, **1**, 1

Yanagita, T., Takahashi, S. and Oinuma, N. (1975d). Drug dependence liability of S-1530 (and nitrazepam) evaluated in the rhesus monkey. *CIEA Preclinical Reports*, **1**, 151

Yanagita, T., Takahashi, S. and Sei, M. (1976). Drug dependence potential of estazolam tested in the rhesus monkey. *CIEA Preclinical Reports*, **2**, 35

Yanagita, T., Wakasa, Y. and Kato, S. (1981c). Dependence potential of alprazolam tested in rhesus monkeys. *CIEA Preclinical Reports*, **7**, 91

Yanagita, T., Wakasa, Y. and Sei, M. (1981d). Dependence potential of clobazam tested in rhesus monkeys. *CIEA Preclinical Reports*, **7**, 115

Yanaura, S. and Tagashira, E. (1975). Dependence on and preference for morphine (II). Comparison among morphine, phenobarbital and diazepam. *Folia Pharmacol. Jpn.*, **71**, 285

Yanaura, S., Tagashira, E. and Suzuki, T. (1975). Physical dependence on morphine phenobarbital and diazepam in rats by drug-admixed food ingestion. *Jpn. J. Pharmacol.*, **25**, 543

Yoshimura, K., Inoue, Y., Sawada, T. and Yamamoto, K. I. (1977). Neuropharmacological studies on drug dependence. (3) Physical dependence on barbiturate-tranquilizer-type drugs in rats. *Jpn. J. Pharmacol.*, **27**, 78P

Yoshimura, K. and Yamamoto, K. I. (1979). Neuropharmacological studies on drug dependence. (1) Effects due to the difference in strain, sex, and drug adminstration time on physical dependence development and characteristics of withdrawal. *Nippon Yakurigaku Zasshi (Folio Pharmacol. Jpn.)*, **75**, 805

Yoshioka, S., Hasegawa, G. and Uno, M. (1970). Zur physischen und psychischen Abhaengigkeit von Meprobamat. Kasuistischer Bericht aus Japan. *Pharmakopsychiat. Neuro-Psychopharmakol.*, **3**, 122–127

Zarco, L. and Almonte, J. (1977). Drug abuse in the Philippines. *Addictive Diseases: an International Journal*, **3**, 1127

Zisook, S. and DeVaul, R. A. (1977). Adverse behavioral effects of benzodiazepines. *Fam. Pract.*, **5**, 963–966

Index

In the subentries of this index, the contraction 'bzd' is used to indicate the term 'benzodiazepines'

absenteeism, alcoholism and 87
abstinence syndrome
  definition viii
  see also withdrawal reactions;
    physical dependence
acquired tolerance *see* tolerance
addiction
  bzd therapy 66–7
  definition viii
agarophobia 101
age and sex, dependence effects 41-2
ageing, anxiety state incidence 84–5
  see also elderly
alcohol
  bzd dependence 42
  medical and social 'costs' 70–1
  open availability 96
  poisoning, mortality 70
  self-medication 102
  tolerance, bzd tolerance relationship
    45
  use and dangers 68, 69
  withdrawal reactions
    barbiturate effects 7
    diazepam effects 17
alcohol type dependence 8, 114
alcoholics
  bzd abuse 55
  post-treatment abstinence, bzd
    therapy 66–7
  tranquillizer dependence 21–3
  tranquillizer tolerance 22
alcoholism
  bzd substitution 87
  bzd therapy 66
  legal aspects 92–9
  mortality 70

amnesia, post-anaesthetic 67
amphetamine type dependence 8
amphetamines
  placebo discrimination 20
  placebo preference rating 19–20
anaesthesia, bzd 67
animal studies
  cross-dependence 14–15, 16–17
  dependence 11–17
  physical dependence 14–17
  primary dependence 14, 15–16
  psychological dependence 11–14
    drug intragastric administration
      14
    drug oral ingestion 12–14
    self-injection 12
  reinforcing properties, bzd 12
  withdrawal reactions 14, 15–16
anorexia nervosa 65
anticonvulsant therapy 67
  long-term bzd therapy 105
antidepressants
  tetracyclic, convulsion threshold
    effects 37, 108
  tricyclic, convulsion threshold
    effects 37, 108, 114
anxiety
  acute, short-term bzd therapy 106
  age-related mean score 85
  bzd therapy indications 62–5
  chronic 100–4
    bzd dependence risks 107
    low-dose intermittent therapy 104
  diagnostic classification (APA) 62,
    64
  DSM-III classification 62, 64
  external environment effects 102–3

159

levels
  bzd intake correlation 25
  tranquillizer use correlation 85–6
performance and 73, 74
physical illness-associated 63–5
rebound 48
recurrence
  bzd withdrawal 35
  difference from withdrawal
    reactions 35–7, 47
  inadequate treatment-induced 35,
    36
sex-related 86–7
withdrawal reaction 34
anxiety states, incidence 84
age effects 84–5
anxiolytics
  environmental changes and 74–5
  long-term use 100–4
    medical surveillance 103–4
    sex relationships 101, 102
    UK 101–2
    USA 102
  method of use 74
  therapy 62–5
  use level justification 84–91
anxious patients, dependence 20–1
ARC I stimulation-euphoria scale,
    diazepam/buspirone
    comparisons 23
asthma, psychosomatic 65
auditory-evoked reactions, EEG,
    withdrawal reactions 38

barbiturate/sedative type dependence 8
barbiturates
  alcohol withdrawal reaction effects 7
  animal primary dependence,
    bezodiazepine differences 15
  bzd receptor affinity 17
  bzd safety comparisons 70
  cross-dependence 16–17
  poisoning, medical and social 'costs'
    71
  reinforcement effect, bzd
    comparisons 14
benzodiazepine abuse 114
  alcoholics 55
  availability relationship 54–5
  'career pathway' 25–6
  primary 49–51
  secondary 51–8
  socio-medical aspects 56–8

withdrawal techniques 55–6
benzodiazepines
  clinical uses 62–8
  CNS binding sites 30
  combinations 83
  dependence 113–14
  intermittent long-term use
    guidelines 108–9
  international availability 62, 63,
    81–2
  legal controls 98–9
    international 98–9
    national 98
  long-acting, withdrawal reactions 48
  long-term use
    continuous, dependence risks 107
    dependence risks 104
    withdrawal 76
  medical and social 'costs' 70–1
  sedative hypnotic use 66
  short-term use guidelines 108
  therapeutic dosage, withdrawal
    reaction incidence 128–33
  use guidelines 108–9
  withdrawal
    follow-up 108–9
    guidelines 109
    management 76–8, 107–8, 114
  see also psychotropics and the various
    types

caffeine, diazepam binding inhibition
    75
caffeine type dependence 8
caffeinism 75
  tobacco smoking association 75
Canada, primary bzd abuse 50
cannabis abuse, 'career pathway' 25–6
cannabis type dependence 8
cardiovascular disorders,
    psychosomatic 65
care/total therapy concept 61, 62, 71
carisprodol, barbiturate cross-
    dependence 16
case reports 116–27
chlordiazepoxide
  barbiturate cross-dependence 16–17
  solution ingestion
    electric shock effects 13
    food deprivation 13
  therapeutic activities 64
  withdrawal reactions 18
chloroquine toxicity, bzd therapy 68

clobazam, therapeutic activities 64
clonazepam, therapeutic activities 64
CNS, benzodiazepine binding sites 30
cocaine type dependence 8
cognitive skills, bzd effects 58
convulsions
    precipitation, antipsychotic drugs 37
    threshold, antidepressant effects 37,
        108, 114
    withdrawal reaction 34, 108, 114
cross-dependence, animal studies
        14–15, 16–17
cross-substitution, alcohol/
        barbiturates 7
crutch phenomenon viii, 46, 48

death, withdrawal reaction 35
dependence
    animal studies 11–17
    anxious patients 20–1
    definition viii
    established, drug withdrawal
        methods 76–8, 107–8
    human studies 18–26
        dependence 26
    medical aspects 72–8
    normal subjects 19–20
pathophysiological mechanisms 30–2
    patterns 27–9
    proneness 27, 48
    receptor change and interaction role
        30
    risks
        bzd long-term continuous therapy
            107
        bzd long-term therapy 104, 113–14
        determination, clinical aspects
            72–3
        low-dose intermittent therapy 104
        reduction 73–5
    therapy-induced 27–8, 114
        dependence levels 72
        differences from abuse 56, 114
        incidence 46–8
        literature update 39–40
    types 7–8
diazepam
    abuse liability 24
    alcohol withdrawal reaction
        reduction 17
    barbiturate cross-dependence 16–17
    binding inhibition, caffeine-induced
        75

cerebral malaria therapy 68
    dosage compliance 73
    euphoriant effect 23
    mood effects 20, 23
    placebo discrimination 20, 23
    placebo preference rating 19–20
    preference, dose-dependent 24
    self-injection studies, rhesus
        monkeys 12
    solution ingestion, water deprivation
        13
    status epilepticus therapy 67
    substitution therapy, bzd
        dependence 76–8
    tetanus therapy 67, 68
    therapeutic activities 64
dopamine, brain turnover, bzd effects
        32
dosage, WHO defined daily dose
        (DDD) 42, 82, 83
drug abuse
    causative factors 94
    control, WHO recommendations
        92–4
    definition viii
    environmental factors 94
    legal aspects 92–9
    management 56–8
    personality factors 94
    product-related factors 94, 95
drug addiction see addiction
drug, definition viii
drug dependence see dependence and
        various types
drug experimenters, bzd abuse 52
drug misuse
    definition viii–ix
    pleasure-seeking 3–7
drug preference, normal subjects 19–20
drug supply
    human rights and 95–6
    legal controls 92–9
        subculture encouragement 97
        therapeutic use restriction 97
        undesirable aspects 97

eclampsia, bzd therapy 68
EEG, withdrawal reactions 38
elderly, anxiolytic long-term use
        relationships 101, 102
    see also age; ageing
elimination rates, withdrawal reactions
        and 45–6

enkephalins, brain turnover, bzd effects 32
environment, external
  drug abuse association 94, 95
  modification 102–3
  anxiolytics and 74–5
ethanol *see* alcohol
Europe, bzd defined daily dose consumption 82, 83
'explosive awakening', rate withdrawal reactions 15

floppy baby syndrome, differences from withdrawal reactions 40
flunitrazepam, therapeutic activities 64
flurazepam, therapeutic activities 64
food deprivation, drug solution substitution 13

GABA-benzodiazepine-chloride channel 30, 31
gastrointestinal disorders, psychosomatic 65

halazepam, euphoriant effect 23
half-life, withdrawal reactions and 33–4
hallucinogen type dependence 8
headaches, psychosomatic 65
heroin, addiction, bzd abuse and 52
5-HIAA, levels, bzd withdrawal 32, 38
HMMA, levels, bzd withdrawal 38
5-HT
  brain turnover, bzd effects 32
  synthesis inhibition, bzd withdrawal and 32
human rights, drug controls and 95–6
human studies, dependence 18–26
  ethical aspects 26
hyeracuity, perceptual changes, withdrawal reaction 34, 36
hyperexcitability, withdrawal reaction 34
hyperthermia, withdrawal reaction 35
hypnotics
  long-term use 105
  use justification 88–90

insomnia
  bzd therapy 66
  long term, 105
  hypnotics use justification 88–90

insomniacs
  dependence 21
  hypnotic preferences 21

legal aspects
  drug control 92–9
  international 92–5
  therapeutic use restriction 97
life stress, tranquillizer use 85–6
limbic system, behavioural inhibition system 32
lorazepam
  dependence 43
    early 46, 48
  placebo preference rating 20
  withdrawal reactions 46, 47, 48
low back pain, psychosomatic 65

malaria, cerebral, diazepam therapy 68
Malaysia, primary bzd abuse 50
mean anxiety score, age-related 85
mental illness, social reactions 79–80
meprobamate, solution ingestion, food deprivation 13
metabolic disorders, psychosomatic 65
methadone
  bzd combination
    drug abuse therapy 57
    euphoric effects 54
  maintenance withdrawal, bzd abuse 52, 53
MOPEG levels, in withdrawal reactions 38
morphine type dependence 8
multiple drug abusers, dependency 23–4
muscle relaxation, long-term bzd therapy 105
muscle spasms, rheumatic disorders, bzd adjuvant therapy 67

narcotics abusers
  bzd abuse incidence 52–3
  bzd use reasons 53–4
narcotics, control, WHO recommendations 92–4
neonates, withdrawal reactions 40
neuromuscular disorders, bzd therapy 67, 105
neurosis, obsessional 101
neurotic disorders, therapy-induced dependence 27

nicotine *see* tobacco smoking
nitrazepam, therapeutic activities 64
noradrenaline, brain turnover, bzd
    effects 32

obsessional neurosis 101
osteoarthritis, muscle spasms, bzd
    adjuvant therapy 67
overdosage 68–71
overeating, compulsive 65
oxazepam
    abuse liability 24
    barbiturate cross-dependence 17
    therapeutic activities 64
oxypertine, bzd withdrawal reaction
    effects 32

panic attacks 100
pentobarbital
    abuse liability 24
    placebo preference rating 20
personality
    dependence-prone 48
    drug abuse-related 94
pharmacotherapy
    effectiveness, psychotherapy
        comparisons 71–2
    psychotherapy combination 65, 66
phenobarbital, substitution therapy,
    bzd withdrawal 77–8, 107–8, 114
phenothiazines, convulsion threshold
    effects 37, 108, 114
Philippines, primary bzd abuse 50
phobic attacks, acute 100
physical dependence 33–8
    animal studies 14–17
    see also cross-dependence;
        withdrawal reactions
physical illness, emotional aspects
    63–5
pleasure-seeking goals 3–7
    good and evil 6–7
    see also socio-recreational abuse
prescribing practices 87–8
primary dependence, animal studies
    14, 15–16
propranolol, bzd withdrawal cover 32,
    108
prostaglandins, brain turnover, bzd
    effects 32
pseudo-dependence 47
psychiatric disorders

consultation rates 84
    incidence 84
    social reactions 79–80
    tranquillizer use 85–6
psychiatric patients, dependence 24–5
psychic distress level, tranquillizer use
    and 85–6
psychic stress, bzd use correlation 101
psychoactive substance, definition ix
    see also psychotropics
psychological dependence
    animal studies 11–14
    clinical aspects 37
    definition ix
    injection timing effects 12
    intravenous self-administration,
        animals 11–12
    oral ingestion studies, animals 12–14
    pleasure-seeking goals 3–7
psychosexual disorders 65
psychosomatic disorders 65
psychotherapy 102
    effectiveness, pharmacotherapy
        comparisons 71–2
    pharmacotherapy combination 65,
        66
psychotropics 4–7
    alcohol use comparisons, Finland
        89, 90
    definition ix
    international control 92–4
    legislation, application variability
        96–7
    rational use education 91
    safety in use 68–71
    scheduling 92–9
    social acceptability 80
    UN definition 4
    1971 convention 93, 95–6, 98–9
    use levels
        decline 81, 83
        population proportion 82–3
        social aspects 80–3

rebound phenomenon 35, 46, 48
    definition x
reinforcing properties,
        benzodiazepines, animal
        studies 12
rheumatoid arthritis, muscle spasms,
        bzd adjuvant therapy 67
Ro 15-1788, withdrawal reaction
        precipitation 16, 31

safety in use 68–71
  therapeutic benefit balance 61
sedative abusers
  benzodiazepine dependence 28
  diazepam/placebo preference 23
  placebo discrimination 22
sedatives
  long-term use 105
  patient selection 106
self-medication 102
sex
  anxiolytic long-term use
    relationships 101, 102
  psychic distress index relationships
    86–7
skin disorders, psychosomatic 65
social class, bzd abuse 51
social problems, bzd use 88–90
socio-recreational abuse 29, 40, 49–58,
    114
  differences from therapeutic
    dependence 56
  see also pleasure-seeking goals
solvent abuse, 'career pathway' 25–6
solvent type dependence 8
status epilepticus, diazepam therapy 67
'street scene', benzodiazepine abuse 29,
    40, 49–58, 114
substitution therapy, withdrawal
    reactions 76–8
Switzerland, primary bzd abuse 50

temazepam, therapeutic activities 64
tetanus, diazepam therapy 67, 68
tetracyclic antidepressants, convulsion
    threshold effects 108
Thailand, primary bzd abuse 50
therapeutic benefit, safety factor
    balance 61
therapeutic regimen, compliance 73
therapy, psychosomatic approach 65
Third World disorders, bzd therapy
    67–8
time interval, bzd withdrawal,
    abstinence reaction 45–6
tobacco
  dependence 8
  open availability 96
tobacco smoking
  caffeinism association 75
  medical and social 'costs' 70–1
  related mortality 70
  use and dangers 68, 69

tolerance 44–5
  definition x
  psychological dependence 37
  receptor change and interaction role
    30, 45
  therapy-induced 27, 28
  to anxiolytic effect 45
  to sedative effect 45
total therapy/care concept 61, 62, 71
tranquillizers
  inappropriate use 90
  misuse 90
  treatment length 90
triazolam
  abuse liability 24
  therapeutic activities 64
tricyclic antidepressants, convulsion
    threshold effects 37, 108, 114

UN
  Commission on Narcotic Drugs 98
  Convention on Psychotropic
    Substances (1971) 93, 95–6,
    98–9
  Declaration of Human Rights 95
uptake patterns 73

water/benzodiazepine solution, animal
    preferences 13
water deprivation, diazepam solution
    substitution 13
WHO
  defined daily dose (DDD) 42, 82, 83
  drug abuse control recommendations
    92–4
  narcotics control recommendations
    92–4
withdrawal reactions 33–8
  alcohol, diazepam effects 17
  animal studies 14, 15–16
  antipsychotic drug therapy 37
  biochemical pathology 38
  chlordiazepoxide 18
  definition x
  differences from floppy baby
    syndrome 40
  differential diagnosis 35–7
  dosage effects 18–19, 42–3
  EEG, auditory evoked potentials 38
  long-acting bzd 48
  management 76–8, 107–8
  narcotics, bzd substitution 53–4

neonates 40
polydrug abuse 78
precipitation, Ro 15-1788 16, 31
propranolol effects 32
pseudo 47
  definition ix
psychological 34
psychopathology 38
psychotic 34–5

rats, 'explosive awakening' 15
rhesus monkeys 15–16
second phase 36
therapeutic dosage, incidence 128–33
time sequence 36
treatment length 19, 42–3, 76

Yerkes-Dodson law, anxiety/
  performance 73, 74